Generation

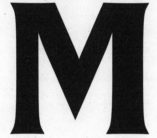

Generation

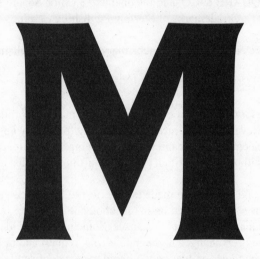

M

LIVING WELL IN PERIMENOPAUSE
AND MENOPAUSE

Dr. Jessica Shepherd
FOREWORD BY DR. JENNIFER ASHTON

**UNION
SQUARE
&CO.**

NEW YORK

UNION
SQUARE
& CO.

NEW YORK

ISBN 978-1-4549-5489-7
ISBN 978-1-4549-5490-3 (e-book)

Library of Congress Control Number: 2024938257

For information about custom editions, special sales, and premium
purchases, please contact specialsales@unionsquareandco.com.

Printed in Canada

2 4 6 8 10 9 7 5 3 1

unionsquareandco.com

Cover design by Catherine Casalino
Cover images by Shutterstock.com: Borisovan.art, Ron Dale, kosmofish,
MURRIRA, Sakarin Sawasdinaka
Interior design by Kevin Ullrich
Image on page 56 courtesy of Wikimedia Commons/Mikael Haggstrom

I dedicate this book to all women—our experiences should be shared instead of silenced. Menopause is a journey, not a race. Through these chapters, I hope you find pieces of yourself that give you the courage to bring heart and understanding to the next segments of your life in wellness.

CONTENTS

Foreword

Menopause is having a moment, with more conversation than ever about this critical stage in a woman's life. This is long overdue and, as the saying goes, better late than never. It is incredible to me that when I, a board-certified OB/GYN, started to experience every possible symptom of perimenopause, I actually did not register or recognize them as such! Instead, my inner dialogue went like this: *I guess this symptom is to be expected at age forty-nine or fifty-one . . .* or *. . . wow, this is annoying, but I really don't have the time to deal with it; I'm too busy . . .* or *. . . I've never had this problem before, but it's not life or death, so I will just ignore it and* *hope it goes away . . .* or *. . . it's not THAT bad; I can handle it.* I had so many head-to-toe symptoms that I didn't connect the dots on them *because* they were so numerous—I definitely didn't imagine that they could *all* be connected with my age and perimenopausal stage. I didn't have the lightbulb moment until a couple of years later, at age fifty-three, when I was working on an article on menopause for my magazine. Holy mother of $@%#!!!!! I had every single symptom and, whether due to denial or stoicism, I hadn't recognize they were symptoms of menopause. Let that sink in. If this can happen to me, it can truly and literally happen to any woman.

But why? There is, in fact, a lot of finger-pointing and blame going on as to why we women are so unprepared for this critical phase in life. Some blame the medical community, others blame our collective mothers, and still others blame society. Personally, I subscribe to the saying that we should be careful when we point a finger (of blame) at someone, because that means that there will be three pointing right back at us. Ultimately, we need to step up and take personal responsibility for what happens to our bodies, and for how we experience what happens. People who go through pregnancy usually make it their business to learn about it, and to learn fast. Menopause should be no different—but for some reason it is. It's time to change that, and waiting until the magical age of fifty is not really an option. An estimated 40 percent of women start experiencing at least one symptom of menopause a full decade before their mid-forties! And lest you think that menopause is just about the hot flash, think again. The most common symptoms include fatigue, joint pain, sleep disturbance, and headaches. And in the workplace, 60 percent of women stated in a recent survey that symptoms of menopause have caused them to rethink their career plans by either considering quitting, retiring, or not seeking a promotion. We have solutions for these symptoms—ignoring them, dismissing them, or suffering in silence is not only unnecessary, it can take a toll physically, psychologically, financially, and socially. But there *is* an answer . . .

Educating ourselves is a process, not a destination, so theoretically it should never end. Every day, we learn new things in medicine and science, and hopefully the increasing amount of research on women's health issues will yield some impactful results. Until then, learning about the spectrum of what may occur during the menopause transition so that you are well prepared for the second half of your life is a great place to start. Happy reading!

Dr. Jennifer Ashton
Board-certified OB/GYN, obesity medicine nutritionist,
and founder of Ajenda
@DrJAshton

Introduction

To exist is to change, to change is
to mature, to mature is to go on
creating oneself endlessly.

—HENRI BERGSON

The Japanese have a term for menopause: konenki. It refers to a period of renewal and reflects the view that women's lives go through many stages. It encourages us to honor the transformations that our bodies, minds, and spirits go through. Each stage of the journey is valuable; each stage is to be treasured.

Change is an inevitable part of the cycle of life, as is aging. How you deal with it is largely up to you. I believe midlife can be a time of empowerment and personal growth. Yes, it brings substantial biological, psychological, social, and emotional changes, especially for women as we go through perimenopause and menopause. I encourage you to, instead of fearing these changes, take ownership of the experience and be an active participant in the journey. When you make the choice to prepare by learning the facts, benefiting from the wisdom of the community, and creating healthy habits, you can optimize how you experience every stage.

More than a million women in America enter menopause each year, and one billion women are anticipated to reach that stage by 2025. Despite these vast numbers, there remains a persistent stigma that prevents women from speaking openly about it. The personal, societal, and economic cost of continuing to push menopause into the background is too high. It is up to us, as proud members of Generation M, to change that.

Historically, menopause has been referred to as "women's hell" or "the death of sex." It is tangled up with negative connotations about women's reproductive health and aging, both taboo subjects in our society. That has led women to internalize the belief that menopause will bring physical changes we can't control and emotional changes that will wreak havoc on our lives. As a woman deep into perimenopause myself and a doctor passionate about advocating for a more equitable and holistic approach to women's health, I refuse to accept that.

Chances are your mother didn't talk to you about menopause. Mine certainly didn't. I know that my mother had a hysterectomy in her forties because of fibroids, but to this day, she is too uncomfortable to speak to me about it in any detail. The message she and so many women of her generation sent, whether they meant to or not, is that menopause is something women must just suffer through; there's nothing we can do about it and there is certainly no reason to talk about such intimate matters.

INTRODUCTION

That left many of us confused about what to expect, in the dark about the very real effects of perimenopause, and puzzled by unanswered questions about the entire transition. One of the reasons I was first drawn to studying women's health was to answer my own questions, and then to use my practice and my platform to educate others.

I always knew I wanted to be a doctor. From a very young age, I was fascinated by how the human body works. In college, I was drawn to courses in human behavior, athletic performance, and nutrition. One day, I started talking to another pre-med student at the gym. Deesha was a few years ahead of me and a star athlete. I began peppering her with questions about her trajectory and she told me that she was majoring in exercise physiology and human sciences. I didn't know that was an option for pre-med students, but I switched my major the next day. This was the track for me, and it opened my eyes to the possibility of combining biology with human behavior.

I spent a year after college working as an exercise physiologist and personal trainer at a cardiac rehabilitation center. One of the first patients I met, Sandra, had never exercised a day in her life. She had high blood pressure and was at a heightened risk for developing diabetes. We worked closely together and each week as she was able to do a bit more, I saw her mood gradually change from fatalistic to optimistic. Within a couple of months, Sandra's cholesterol, blood pressure, and weight had all improved. Just as important, she had a newfound sense of confidence. That experience confirmed my belief that a holistic approach that includes exercise, nutrition, and psychology is the best way to improve patients' physical and emotional health. That has been my guiding principle ever since.

INTRODUCTION

When I started medical school the following year, I was determined to dive deeper into the science that would allow me to combine cutting-edge medicine with this body/mind/spirit approach. I have always loved babies and thought at first that I would be an obstetrician. As I got deeper into my studies, though, I realized that I was interested in the *entire* spectrum of women's health, not just pregnancy. I was shocked by how little attention was being paid to gynecological health beyond the reproductive years. You would think that menopause—which, remember, affects 50 percent of the human race—would get more than a single chapter in a textbook, but it didn't. In fact, throughout medical school, we spent approximately eight hours on the entire menopausal transition.

We were taught the basic facts, that estrogen decreases and women get hot flashes, but that was pretty much it. There was no discussion about the vast array of emotional, sexual, and psychological changes women go through. Perimenopause was barely mentioned at all. Women's stories were not being heard, and the research dollars were going elsewhere. The result was a generation of doctors who were not given the necessary information to help women mitigate symptoms, lower disease risks, or improve their quality of life. Frankly, that drove me mad and led to my passion to do everything I could to help change it.

Women's health, through adolescence, pregnancy, menopause, and aging, has been put on the back burner for centuries. That not only fails women, it fails society at large. Women are so often at the center of their families. We comprise half the workforce in this country. If we are not functioning at our best, it has a negative impact on the people in our lives, from family members to employers. It behooves us to think of menopause as so much more than a "woman's" issue.

It is just as important to recognize the long history of racial disparities in health care in the United States. Recent studies have pointed out the large variations between African American, Hispanic, Japanese, Chinese, and Caucasian women when it comes to the severity of their symptoms and the treatment options they are offered. Education, financial strain, family history, and health habits also impact menopause. None of this was taught in medical school. As a Black female physician and menopause expert, I am dedicated to ensuring that when we talk about menopause, *all* women are included.

Fast forward to my initial interactions with patients while I was doing my residency in OB/GYN at Drexel University–Hahnemann Hospital in Philadelphia and quickly saw the real-life effects of this systemic avoidance of the intricacies of menopause. One morning, a woman named Carol came into the clinic where I was working, complaining of horrific night sweats. She couldn't remember the last time she slept through the night, and she was clearly depressed. In a whisper, she confided she had also lost all interest in sex. The doctor she had seen before had asked her about hot flashes but nothing more. She was left to assume her loss of libido was due to some failing on her part rather than a common response to fluctuating hormones. At the time, there weren't many treatment options to offer. The research into menopause in general, and hormone replacement therapy specifically, was sparse and often misleading. While I assured Carol that what she was going through was completely normal, I wanted better answers for her, and for all women entering this stage of life. Myself included.

We have made progress since those days, but not enough. As a society, we remain largely uncomfortable speaking about women's reproductive health in general and menopause in particular. The cloud of embarrassment and shame that surrounds the topic has led to gaps in awareness, education, and advocacy. It prevents women from being able to make informed decisions based on the latest research, and benefit from the full range of medical and lifestyle options now open to us.

As you will learn in the pages that follow, having a sense of purpose is one of the key elements of both emotional and physical health. My own purpose is to champion the discussion around this time of women's lives and help us all push past limiting beliefs into a future where women feel powerful, sexy, and valued no matter their age.

Too many women are still embarrassed to talk openly about perimenopause and menopause. The sense of being alone, and the silence it leads to, can prevent you from learning about the symptoms, treatment options, and lifestyle changes that can help you feel your best, have more energy, experience better sleep, enjoy satisfying sex, lower your risk of certain diseases, and have a stronger sense of self. The more you can use this knowledge to prepare, whether you are in your thirties, forties, fifties, or beyond, the better you will be able to face the future from a place of physical and emotional strength.

That is the work we are here to do together.

Own Your Journey

As overall health improves and life expectancy increases, most women can expect to live 40 percent of their life after menopause. That is a powerful incentive to take control of your health now. Owning your menopause journey by implementing the concrete positive steps you will find here not only will help you feel empowered, but can lessen symptoms and improve your quality of life for all the years that follow.

Stop for a minute and ask yourself: *When I look at my future, how do I want to feel? What can I do today to set myself up for a healthier tomorrow?* These are the questions we are here to answer.

There is no one-size-fits-all solution. Rather, the most successful strategy for thriving through perimenopause, menopause, and aging in general includes small adjustments to your lifestyle habits such as exercise, nutrition, psychological practices, mindfulness, and medication. This whole-life approach is particularly important when it comes to dealing with hormonal transitions, because the symptoms themselves are so interrelated. Here's just one example: hot flashes can interrupt sleep. Interrupted sleep can make weight gain more likely. Weight gain can put you at higher risk for certain diseases. The good news is that just as there is a cascade effect with symptoms, there are ways to interrupt the cycle. Exercise can help improve sleep and weight gain. Stress-reducing techniques can improve brain and physical health.

Throughout this book, you will learn how to make the small changes that have a big impact on virtually every area of your life and health. These are realistic, actionable steps you can fold into your diet, fitness, and lifestyle routine. Steps that you choose. Steps that you can stick with. Steps that will enable you to become the CEO of your own health.

Research published by the *British Journal of General Practice* shows that it takes ten weeks to build a new habit, and the best way to make the habit stick is through small incremental changes. For you, that might mean building five minutes of breath work into your day, adding more protein to your diet, or learning to recognize and change negative self-talk. In this book, you will find specific ways to do just that and more, and you can return to these pages again and again, continually adding more building blocks to your repertoire.

It will take practice. Society sends women going through perimenopause and menopause the message that our value diminishes after our reproductive years. It can be hard not to internalize those wrongheaded beliefs and devalue ourselves. I truly believe, though, that each positive step you take will lead you to a new sense of agency and the confidence to write your own narrative.

Welcome to Generation M!

As a doctor, a sister, a friend, a community leader, and a mother, I know we are stronger together. Not only will I give you the information that will help you understand what is happening to your body, but I'll introduce you to experts in fitness, nutrition, meditation, intimacy, and healthy aging who will share their wisdom and practical tips. You will find answers to some of the most common questions, and you'll hear from women like you about their personal challenges and the secrets of what worked for them throughout their own perimenopause and menopause journey.

It is never too early—or too late—to start creating the healthy habits that will help you face the future with strength and confidence. And I will be by your side every step of the way.

Shall we begin?

The Secret to Building Healthy Habits That Last

The *British Journal of General Practice* has studied the most effective route to positive change. They recommend the following steps to building healthy habits. You can apply it to all the building blocks you will find throughout this book, but let's use incorporating more steps into your day as an example.

1. **Decide on a goal that you would like to achieve for your health.** One of the keys to successful habit formation is to make sure your goal is realistic. You've probably heard that taking 10,000 steps a day is the ideal amount for optimal health. That's great, but the latest research also shows that as few as 3,000 to 4,000 steps per day can lower your risk of cardiovascular disease and overall mortality. For most people, that takes just about thirty minutes. Totally doable, right?

2. **Choose a simple action that you can do on a daily basis and will get you moving toward your goal.** For many women with busy lives that include taking care of kids and the home, and holding down a job, even thirty minutes can be hard to come by. Instead of giving up on days when you can't find that block of time, commit to breaking it up into five- or ten-minute increments. If you have a fitness tracker, set it to remind you to move. You can also set the timer on your phone to prompt you to get up every hour, even if it is just to walk around your home or office. Remember, anything you do is better than nothing.

3. **Plan when and where you will do your chosen action.**
   Don't leave adding steps to chance. Make the decision
   ahead of time that when you drive to work or go shopping,
   you will park your car farther away than you do now. If
   you live in the city and take public transportation, plan
   on getting out a stop before you normally do and walking
   the rest of the way. When your schedule allows, start or
   end your day with a fifteen-minute walk around your
   neighborhood. Write it into your calendar as you would
   any other appointment to help you prioritize it.

4. **Pair the desired action with something you already
   do.** One easy way to get more steps in is to pace whenever
   you are on a phone call. You can do the walk-and-talk at
   home (no one has to know if you are simply circling the
   living room!), or, if feasible, step outside at work for a few
   minutes. Set aside a walk as your time to return calls. By
   marrying the two activities, you increase the likelihood
   that you will stick with it.

5. **It will get easier with time, and within ten weeks you
   should find you are doing it automatically without
   even having to think about it.** Because you have broken
   your goal up into manageable increments, it will be
   easier for the additional steps to become a natural part of
   your day.

6. **Congratulations, you've made a healthy habit!**

CHAPTER ONE

Your Roadmap: Where Are You Now? Where Are You Going?

> We cannot change what we are not
> aware of, and once we are aware,
> we cannot help but change.
>
> —SHERYL SANDBERG

Gwendolyne Osbourne was forty-four when she started to experience unusually heavy periods. "At first, I tried to ignore it," she says. "I couldn't sleep and everything got on my nerves. I have three kids at home and I was going through a lot of upheaval in my personal and professional life. I didn't talk to my doctor about my symptoms because I assumed I was too young to be experiencing hormonal changes. It was only when I began getting so hot at night that I had to strip off my pajamas that I started to put it together. People tell you about childbirth, but no one warned me about perimenopause. I had no idea what to expect, much less who to turn to for advice. Now the only thing I want to know is how long is this going to last?"

I talk to so many women like Gwendolyne who are confused about where they are in their perimenopause and menopause journey. Even the most health-conscious, informed women look at me with confusion in their eyes and ask: *How do I know where I am in the transition? Why do I feel like I have lost control of my body? When will it stop?*

That sense of helplessness is understandable. Not only has there been a decided lack of clear information—and, worse, too much out-dated information—but the experience itself is vastly different for every woman. We tend to want binary answers in life. Yes or no. In or out. Start or finish. We expect a firm diagnosis from doctors. But menopause is more complicated than that. Perimenopause, menopause, and postmenopause do not have hard-and-fast boundaries. Instead, the hormonal transition is more like an ongoing symphony, with ups and downs, peaks and valleys.

No two women will experience menopause at the same time in the same way. As we will see, race, ethnicity, genetics, and lifestyle all influence the transition. Along the way, your hormones, and the physical, psychological, and emotional upheavals they cause, will ebb and flow from your first period until years after your last. It is not a straight line, which can make it hard to decipher where exactly you are in your personal transition. For instance, you may still be having regular periods but have other symptoms, like brain fog, that place you squarely in perimenopause. You may assume that you are too young to be going through menopause despite having increasingly frequent hot flashes. This might lead you to dismiss your symptoms or think you have to suffer in silence. That can keep you from getting the help you need in a timely fashion.

My own sister, Desiree, never realized her achy joints were due to her low level of estrogen until she went on hormone replacement therapy (HRT)[1] and suddenly it didn't hurt to get out of bed in the morning. One of my patients, Helena, assumed her frequent headaches were due to a stressful job until I asked her to track her periods and she realized they were three months apart. She had no idea that headaches can be caused by decreasing estrogen.

While hot flashes get all the attention, there are in fact twenty (!) symptoms related to perimenopause and menopause. These might include irregular or heavy periods, hot flashes, irritability, sleep disturbances, low libido, or brain fog. It is even more confusing because so many of the symptoms, from insomnia to anxiety, can be caused or exacerbated by life events. Social media and society at large are permeated by such a negative take on menopause that the result can be a sense of helplessness when it comes to dealing with symptoms. Rather than giving in to this negative mindset, arming yourself with solid information not only will help you make lifestyle tweaks that can lessen the impact of symptoms, but also can bring a much-needed sense of agency and yes, even optimism.

---

1   Throughout this book I will continue to use the acronym HRT for hormone replacement therapy. In other sources, including some of the research I cite, it has come to be referred to as menopausal hormone therapy (MHT). I believe they are essentially the same and will continue to use HRT for the sake of clarity.

BUILDING BLOCK
Your Symptom Checklist

Talk to your doctor if you have four or more of these symptoms, or if symptoms go on for longer than four months. There is a good chance they are related to changes in your fluctuating estrogen levels that begin during perimenopause as ovarian follicles begin to wane.

- Changes in your menstrual cycle including skipped and/or irregular periods, or bleeding that is heavier or lighter than usual

- Mood swings, including anxiety, depression, and irritability

- Feeling disconnected from your body physically and emotionally

- Problems with memory, concentration, and brain fog

- Headaches or migraines

- Hot flashes

- Skin conditions, including dryness and acne

- Difficulty sleeping

- Night sweats

- Heart palpitations

- Recurrent urinary tract infections (UTIs)

- Vaginal dryness and pain

- Reduced sex drive

- Discomfort during sex

- Change in ability to orgasm

- Hair loss or thinning

- Increase in facial hair

- Joint stiffness, aches, and pains

- Dry, thinning skin

- Tinnitus

The first step is to keep a list of all your symptoms and bring it in to your doctor to start a discussion. Because symptoms can wax and wane, this running list will help provide a record of what you have been experiencing over a period of months. If your doctor doesn't ask about symptoms, make sure you bring them up anyway and explain what you are experiencing. That will provide clues about how and when you might benefit from treatments, including hormone replacement therapy, and the lifestyle changes that can make a huge difference in how you experience both perimenopause and menopause.

The Generation M Journey: An Overview

Before we delve into each stage of the menopausal transition, its symptoms, and the proactive steps you can take to lessen the impact, it will help to have an overview of the entire process from birth through your reproductive to post-reproductive years.

Every female is born with the entire number of ovarian follicles they will have throughout their life. In utero, a female has approximately five million follicles. By the time she's born, that number has gone down to two million. During menstruation, the brain releases a hormone that tells the ovary to produce estrogen. When estrogen peaks, the follicle will release an egg. If the egg is fertilized, estrogen will level off while progesterone rises to support pregnancy. There's a beautiful precise timing to this cadence.

Over time, the number of ovarian follicles begins to wane, which reduces the production of estradiol, the most active form of estrogen. You may not notice it at first, but as your reserve of ovarian follicles

Q: Should I have my hormones checked to find out where I am in the journey?

A: For most women, hormone tests done during perimenopause are of limited use because of the range of hormonal fluctuations that occur throughout your cycle. They could show completely different hormone levels within a one-month span. Tracking symptoms and missed periods can be enough to tell whether you are in perimenopause. If you are experiencing bothersome menopausal symptoms, it can be appropriate to start hormone replacement therapy regardless of what your blood work shows, though a number of other considerations should be weighed into your decision. (See Chapter 4, "The ABCs of HRT," for more information on HRT.) That said, your doctor may want to consider running a blood panel for a baseline picture or to rule out any medical conditions. For women who have had hysterectomies but still have their ovaries, and thus can't use menstrual bleeding as an indicator, testing hormone levels every six months can be useful. Lab tests typically measure follicle-stimulating hormone (FSH) levels, which start to increase when you get closer to the menopausal phase. When a woman's FSH blood level is consistently elevated to thirty or higher and she has not had a menstrual cycle for a year, it is generally accepted that she has reached menopause. As with all medical advice, check with your own doctor before making any decisions.

depletes, you will begin to experience fluctuations in estrogen levels, which can cause heavy or irregular periods, mood swings, and a host of other changes. One of estrogen's other jobs is to regulate your body temperature. That's why dropping estrogen levels can result in hot flashes, often one of the first symptoms of perimenopause.

Your body will try to compensate for the lack of estrogen by increasing the amount of the hormone that stimulates the growth of eggs in the ovaries. This follicle-stimulating hormone (FSH) works to help your body maintain its menstrual cycles. A high FSH level indicates that your body is no longer producing enough estrogen. When the follicles are fully depleted, your periods stop.

The Three Stages:
The Preseason, the Main Event,
the After-Party

Here's a snapshot of the hormonal ebb and flow from perimenopause to postmenopause.

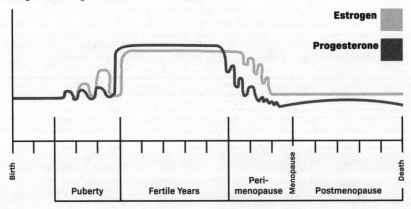

Stages of Menopause

Understanding the changes in your body during menopause.

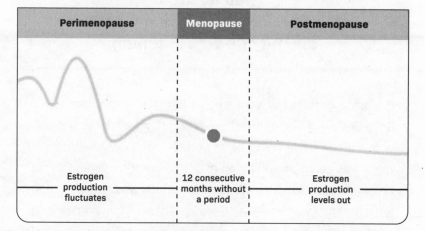

STAGE 1	STAGE 2	STAGE 3
Perimenopause	**Menopause**	**Postmenopause**

Estrogen production fluctuates — 12 consecutive months without a period — Estrogen production levels out

Perimenopause: The Preseason

What's happening:
You are coming out of the reproductive phase of life as ovarian follicles get depleted and estrogen wanes.

Average age:
Forty-seven, though it can begin in your early, mid-, or late forties. Results from cross-sectional studies have indicated that the first endocrine changes characteristic of the onset of perimenopause may begin at around age forty-five.

Average duration:
Four years

Menopause: The Main Event

What's happening:
Technically, natural (i.e., non–medically or surgically induced) menopause is a one-day event, indicating that you have gone twelve months without a period. Estrogen levels fluctuate but are increasingly low, or undetectable.

Average age:
The average age ranges from about forty-nine to fifty-one years old, depending on ethnicity. Black, Asian, and Latina women on average begin menopause earlier than white women.

Duration: One day.

Postmenopause: The After-Party

What's happening:
While everything after the twelve-month mark of menstrual cessation is clinically considered postmenopausal, we will use the term instead to refer to the time when the most severe symptoms wane or stop.

Duration:
Hot flashes resulting from menopause last an average of 4.8 years for Japanese women, 5.4 years for Chinese women, 6.5 years for white women, 8.9 years for Hispanic women, and 10.1 years for Black women.

MELANIE'S STORY

I had no idea what was going on with my body— and no one was listening.

I started getting hot flashes and night sweats when I was thirty-nine. It wasn't that long after I had a child, so it didn't occur to me that I might be in perimenopause. I knew something was going on and I tried to talk to my doctor about it, but he didn't really hear me. We both assumed I was too young and left it at that. I was confused because I had no explanation, and frustrated because I didn't feel I was being taken seriously. I didn't talk about it with my friends because I thought I was the only one going through this experience.

By the time I was forty-three, I was anxious all the time. I had trouble sleeping and I started having panic attacks, which I had never had before. I was getting hot flashes at work and had trouble remembering things. I ended up going into menopause by forty-five, which was much earlier than I expected.

That's when I found a new doctor who really listened to me, and we started talking about solutions. At first, I was worried about taking hormones because of the side effects they might have. What tipped the decision for me was that I found out I have osteopenia, early-stage osteoporosis, and I learned that estrogen replacement can help protect my bones. Once I started HRT, I felt so much better. I began sleeping again, my confidence came back, and my anxiety lessened. The hot flashes aren't completely gone, but they're better.

If I had been more knowledgeable about symptoms or had been a better advocate for myself, I could have gotten help sooner. I've learned to listen to my body and pay closer attention to what it needs in terms of nutrition and exercise. Most important, I've become a much better advocate for myself, which has given me greater confidence in all areas of my life. Honestly, I feel freer to be myself.

—Melanie Ross Mills, 51

The decline in estrogen affects much more than your menstrual cycle or the sudden onset of hot flashes that put global warming to shame. It has far-ranging implications for your health. Because there are estrogen receptors—the proteins in cells that kick estrogen into action—all over your body, virtually every organ, from your brain to your bladder, is affected when the hormone dips.

The loss of estrogen increases the risk of heart disease, the number one killer of women in America. It decreases calcium absorption in the bones that can lead to osteoporosis. Lower estrogen levels have also been associated with weight gain and obesity, vaginal dryness, lowered libido, depression, and sleep disturbances. I realize that sounds overwhelming, if not downright depressing. Keep in mind that not everyone experiences *all* of these things. And you have agency to fight back. In the coming chapters, you will find ways to address each of these changes, including HRT and simple, actionable lifestyle tweaks that can go a long way to offset disease risk. I'm not saying menopause is fun. What I *am* saying is that you have choices.

CHAPTER TWO

The Preseason: Perimenopause

The best preparation for tomorrow is doing your best today.

—H. JACKSON BROWN JR.,
P.S. I LOVE YOU

S uddenly you're waking up five times a night, you're snapping at your dog, and your jeans seem to have shrunk three inches. But you're only in your forties. Plus, you are still getting your period regularly. What gives?

Welcome to the preseason.

Despite the fact that one billion women around the world will experience perimenopause by 2025, and most will be in their forties, far too little focus, if any at all, has been put on this sometimes-baffling time of life. That is unfortunate, not least because perimenopause is the perfect opportunity to prime your body and your mind for what's to come. After all, you wouldn't run a marathon without training first, right? Building healthy habits now not only will ease perimenopause, but also can keep symptoms from worsening when the Main Event hits, and protect your health long after menopause.

The average age for the onset of perimenopause is forty-seven, and it generally lasts about four years, but there are huge variations in both the start date and duration due to family history, ethnicity, lifestyle, and genetics. It is entirely possible to have no changes to your menstrual cycle but be in the middle of a meeting when it suddenly feels as if there's a heat lamp aimed directly at your face. Perhaps your perfectly charming partner makes you want to gnash your teeth just for saying good morning. Because this is a time of life when many women are balancing kids, jobs, and older parents, it can be hard to tell what is causing the symptoms. Are you stressed because of your hormones? Because of everything you are dealing with? All of the above?

While poor sleep, weight gain, and fatigue are often a natural result of getting older that everyone experiences, for women, hormonal shifts can exacerbate the symptoms. The truth is, it's not always possible to tease apart the cause. Aging and menopause are inextricably linked. Because the range of ages when women go through perimenopause varies widely, it is important to bring up any symptoms to your doctor, even if they don't ask. You don't want to miss out on the positive steps you can take now to treat the symptoms and improve your quality of life.

BUILDING BLOCK
How to Find the Right Doctor

Because the symptoms of perimenopause can be hard to pinpoint, it may be tempting to try to ignore them or feel they are not worth bringing up to your doctor. They are! Pay attention to your body, keep your checklist going, and bring it with you to appointments. If you feel your doctor is not listening, ask your friends for a recommendation or do online research to find a doctor well-versed in menopause, not just in childbirth. It is especially important to see a doctor who can provide up-to-date information on HRT, and clearly explain the pros and cons to you. The North American Menopause Society has a database on their website to help you find a menopause practitioner in your area. See https://portal.menopause.org.

The Dimmer Switch

Perimenopause is akin to a dimmer switch slowly lowering as estrogen levels start dialing down and you get closer to menopause. During your forties, fluctuations in the hormones that regulate estrogen, along with a decrease in testosterone (yes, women have testosterone, too), can impact your energy levels, mood, weight distribution, and even your cholesterol makeup. You may not be aware of the changes at first, but gradually they will become more frequent until you can't help but notice them.

At the start of perimenopause, your periods will still be pretty regular and symptoms will be infrequent. You may start to notice a change in your sleep patterns, but in many instances the symptoms are not consistent, and may not be severe. It's estimated that 30 to 70 percent of perimenopausal women get hot flashes, and they are likely to be mild in nature at these earlier stages. But don't get used to that—chances are, they will increase in frequency and severity.

Vaginal symptoms, including dryness and pain during sex, can start relatively early in the transition. Unlike hot flashes, which tend to improve as you move past menopause, vaginal dryness does not get better without treatment. It is one of the reasons it can be beneficial to begin hormone replacement therapy (HRT) *before* you reach menopause.

As perimenopause progresses, estrogen levels will continue to drop. The late transition is marked by at least two missed periods in a row, but because periods can be wildly irregular, even figuring that out can be confusing. Kelly Ripa shared her experience with this on her podcast, *Let's Talk Off Camera.* "I could barely sit up and I was like, 'I don't know what's wrong with me,' and [my doctor] said, 'You're probably perimenopausal' and I was like 'No, I get my period constantly' and she said, 'Yeah that's perimenopause. That's part of it.'"

The heavy periods that some women experience during perimenopause are due to hormonal fluctuations that cause estrogen to spike without sufficient progesterone to balance it. This can lead to changes in the wall of the uterus, resulting in excessive bleeding. The situation tends to resolve once you hit menopause. Because heavy bleeding can make you more prone to anemia, talk to your doctor if you are experiencing this. They may recommend changes in diet and/or a multivitamin with iron.

Uterine fibroids, growths in the uterus that are usually benign, also tend to peak during perimenopause. They are three times more common in Black women and two times more common in Hispanic women compared to white women. While there is no single answer that explains this discrepancy, a diet lower in fruits and vegetables, environmental factors such as the chemicals in hair relaxers, and higher levels of stress are thought to play a role.

Fibroids can lead to heavy bleeding and pain, and they can put added pressure on your bladder. Your doctor can diagnose fibroids through a number of methods, including a pelvic exam, sonogram, or MRI. A diagnosis can tell you how many fibroids you have and their size, and it can lead to a recommendation from your doctor about whether you should consider treatment options. Whether or not you seek treatment for fibroids depends on the amount of bleeding you are experiencing and how close you are to menopause, when heavy bleeding from fibroids usually subsides. Some of the treatment options include progesterone injections, like an IUD that releases progesterone, or gonadotropin-releasing hormone (GnRH) agonists and antagonists that decrease both estrogen and progesterone levels to shrink fibroids and reduce uterine bleeding. It may also be possible to have a surgical myomectomy, which can remove fibroids while keeping the uterus intact. For some women, an endometrial ablation that destroys the lining of the uterus to stop bleeding is an option. Finally, a hysterectomy that removes your uterus is sometimes recommended, particularly for women with large or multiple fibroids. Each option has different risk factors and recovery time. (See Chapter 3: "The Main Event and the After-Party: Menopause and Postmenopause" for more about surgically and medically induced menopause, including the racial disparities in how treatment is delivered.)

When you go twelve months without menstruation, you are out of the perimenopause woods and officially in menopause. Night sweats and hot flashes may begin, or increase in severity and frequency, if they haven't already, which can further disrupt sleep. Around this time, weight often begins to accumulate around your middle and brain fog becomes more common. We will examine a range of ways to mitigate these symptoms in upcoming chapters.

Preseason Training: Prepare Your Body, Mind, and Spirit

Because perimenopause has received so little attention, it's easy to assume there is little you can or should do at this stage to mitigate

Q: Can I still get pregnant?

A: The short answer is yes. While getting pregnant is certainly less likely and continues to decline after the age of forty, if you are not planning on having a baby, it is important to use birth control. While the risk of pregnancy is low, it's not impossible. Women over forty give birth to 4 percent of all babies; 75 percent of those are unplanned, in part because many women assume they can no longer get pregnant. Many women in perimenopause ovulate more than once a month, which can also make it harder to predict fertility.

Oral contraceptives can be used safely by healthy non-smoking women until their mid-fifties, but talk to your doctor about the risks versus the benefits of using oral contraceptives after the age of thirty-five.

symptoms. Nothing could be further from the truth. By taking positive steps now, you will set yourself up to better weather the hormonal storms of menopause, lessen your risk of certain diseases, maintain your weight, and deal with a decrease in libido.

There is a common misconception that HRT is meant only for women in menopause. In fact, starting HRT during perimenopause not only can help lessen current symptoms, including hot flashes, mood swings, and trouble sleeping, but also can reduce their severity once you hit menopause. (Consider it a form of future-proofing your body.) We will do a deep dive on HRT shortly (see Chapter 4), but I want to emphasize the window of opportunity that perimenopause presents to ensure you discuss the options with your doctor *before* menopause.

Here's a quick snapshot of the benefits of starting HRT during perimenopause: It can reduce the chances of depression and combat vaginal dryness. It can help prevent osteoporosis and heart disease. And, if that's not enough, HRT's ability to help prevent Alzheimer's disease is strongest when it is begun during perimenopause.

Prep for the Pause:
Five Steps to Take Now

Rather than viewing perimenopause as the waiting room for the Main Event (menopause), I encourage you to establish habits as soon as possible, hopefully in your early forties, to ease your entire transition. Whether or not you decide to take HRT, tweaking your lifestyle (we're not talking about a major overhaul) will set you up to be stronger, both emotionally and physically. That's an investment in your future worth making. We will go into these steps in more detail in later chapters. Here are five to consider *now*.

1. **Track your cycles.** Menopause officially begins when you go twelve months without a period, but it can be hard to remember when your last period was. Use an app or calendar to keep track.

2. **Establish a sleep routine.** Loss of sleep not only leaves you less able to deal with daily stresses, but also has a direct impact on weight, disease risk, and longevity. Now is the time to set up bedtime rituals that will help you get the necessary shut-eye. (See Chapter 5, "Will I Ever Sleep Again?")

3. **Mind your muscles.** Decreasing hormone levels can lead to a loss of lean muscle. Adding more protein to your diet and beginning weight training can help curb your appetite, maintain your weight, and protect your bones. (See Chapter 7, "Weight, What?" and Chapter 8, "The Exercise Rx.")

4. **Begin a meditation practice.** Too little attention is paid to the emotional changes perimenopause can bring, including an increase in anxiety and depression. Meditation can decrease stress (which is bound to happen) and help you sleep. That brain fog that you suddenly find yourself lost in? It helps with that, too.

5. **Don't keep it to yourself.** When you are going through the emotional swings of perimenopause, it can be tempting to shut yourself off from others, but that will only make the experience harder. Isolation also puts you at greater risk for depression. Sharing what you are going through with friends will give them a chance to commiserate, and maybe do some venting of their own. (See Chapter 10, "This Is Your Brain on Menopause," for more ways to stay connected.)

BUILDING BLOCK

Five Simple Steps to Building a Meditation Practice

One of the first symptoms of perimenopause I experienced was trouble focusing. I had tried meditation on and off but had never been that disciplined about it. I knew all the research that shows how it can help with mental clarity, and I recommitted to making it part of my life. I'll be honest: I'm still working on making it a habit. (I have building blocks to work on, too.) I am a big believer in learning from other women, so I turned to my friend Christiane Wolf, MD, PhD, who is not only a gynecologist but also a meditation teacher and the author of *A Clinician's Guide to Teaching Mindfulness,* for advice. She has been generous enough to share her tips for beginning a meditation practice.

1. Protect your time and space.

- You will greatly enhance your sense of safety by making sure you won't be interrupted while you meditate.
- Let your partner, kids, roommates, or colleagues know that your meditation time is off-limits.
- Put your phone on mute (unless you use it to listen to a meditation app). Put it far away if it vibrates whenever a text or email comes in.
- Make a decision about your pets. A lot of pets love when you meditate and are happy to snuggle with you or on you when you meditate. If you like that, cool. If not, ship them out during that time.

2. Find a place that makes you feel safe and comfortable.

- What helps you to feel safe in your body and in your environment while meditating?
- If you are not sure, you might want to try various locations in the room and pay close attention to what your body is telling you. Safe? Safer? Not so much?

3. Create a space that is dedicated to meditation.

- You could set your chair in a way that you look out of the window or glass door into the garden.
- Or set up a little table or shelf. On it put some things that inspire you: a photograph, a framed quotation, flowers, etc.

4. Choose a comfortable sitting posture.

- Make sure that your sitting posture is so comfortable that you can hold it for the time of your meditation without the need to move or shift.
- You can sit on a chair or on the mat or even lie down on the floor, but you need to find a posture that signifies dignity and ease for you.

5. Create a routine.

- Practice at the same time of the day.
- Create a pre-meditation routine (a cup of tea, for example).
- Experiment with reading something related to meditation for five minutes.
- Do a little ritual, like lighting a candle or nice incense stick or sounding a bell (it is struck three times, traditionally).
- Assume the same body posture.

BLAKE'S STORY

Perimenopause was THE LAST thing I expected.

I was going through a rough time in my mid-forties, including a divorce, a high-pressure career, and raising kids. I've never had to diet and suddenly I gained thirty pounds, which made me feel miserable. I was irritable, I had no interest in sex, and I wasn't sleeping. I just attributed it to getting older and life in general. It didn't occur to me that it might be related to hormones until I was about to go on a trip.

I packed white jeans and all these sundresses. Suddenly I got the heaviest period I had ever had. I was totally unprepared because I'd just had my period two weeks before. That's when it all began to fit together. Yes, the changes were due to what was going on in my life and getting older, but I was also well into perimenopause.

Knowing what was going on put me in a much better place. I realized I had to change my diet and start exercising, which I had let slip. It didn't happen overnight, but understanding that

I didn't have to be at the mercy of my hormones spurred me to keep at it. I felt more in control, which boosted my self-esteem and helped me stick with it.

One of the things that really helped me was beginning to meditate. I only do it for ten minutes, three or four times a week, but it's made me better able to deal with outside distraction and reduce my stress levels. When I can't sleep, I turn on a guided meditation.

Now, two years later, I've dropped the weight and started dating. I made a conscious decision to be open about all the changes I'm going through, whether it's hot flashes or mood swings, with my new partner. It was hard at first, but it has led to a deeper relationship. Besides, sometimes you just have to laugh about waking up drenched.

—Blake Stephenson, 53

CHAPTER THREE

The Main Event and the After-Party: Menopause and Postmenopause

My mission in life is not merely to survive,
but to thrive and do so with some
passion, some compassion, some
humor, and some style.

—MAYA ANGELOU

Menopause is a natural stage of life, just as puberty is. Both can be turbulent. Both affect virtually every aspect of your body, mood, and psyche. Puberty, though, is seen as a rite of passage celebrated by most cultures, from Sweet Sixteen parties to quinceañeras and bar and bat mitzvahs. Puberty may be messy, but it is accepted as the doorway to the fullness of adulthood.

Unfortunately, the historic view of patriarchy has framed menopause strictly in negative terms, giving women the message that once our reproductive years are over, we are no longer useful, attractive, or even of interest.

That is, quite frankly, ridiculous.

I refuse to accept the premise that menopause is the end of vitality. Generation M is not about to go slinking quietly off into the sunset prematurely. Instead, I urge you to change that outdated script and think of it as the entry point to the rest of your life. Your birth day. Your reset day.

Remember, most of us can expect to live 40 percent of our lives postmenopause. You get to decide what you want that to look and feel like. I, for one, vote for heading into the next stage knowing that I have done everything I can to move forward from a place of strength—physically, mentally, and spiritually.

The actions you take now will go a long way to making a vibrant second half of life a reality. I'm not naïve enough to think there won't be challenges and occasional rough patches, for me and for you. The very real changes that menopause brings, from brain fog to lowered libido, cannot be wished away. Along with the immediate symptoms—hello, hot flashes—the loss of estrogen also has long-term implications, including an elevated risk of heart disease and osteoporosis. That doesn't mean you should just throw up your hands and wait for the inevitable. Whether or not you decide to use HRT, there is strong research showing that practices such as yoga, mindfulness, breath work, and acupuncture can provide relief for a range of symptoms, including insomnia, anxiety, and yes, even hot flashes. There are specific exercise and nutritional tips that can slash your disease risk. We'll get into all of them.

The One–Day Kickoff to the Rest of Your Life

Let's start by defining what menopause actually is. Clinically speaking, natural (i.e., not medically induced) menopause is the single day that marks twelve months without a period. The average age for its onset is fifty-one for white women in the United States and forty-nine for Black women. Hispanic and Native American women also tend to hit menopause earlier than white women, while Japanese women tend to go through menopause later. These are just averages, though. Many factors influence when menopause begins, including family history, genetics, weight, and lifestyle. Smoking, drinking, and a lack of exercise can all contribute to an earlier menopause. While it is not a one-for-one predictor, the age your mother went through menopause can also offer you a clue about what to expect.

You are technically postmenopausal after the day you hit natural menopause, but because it is an ongoing transition, I am going to talk about menopause as the years in which you are no longer menstruating and symptoms are at their height. Symptoms tend to be most prevalent and severe during the first one to two years and then slowly begin to wane. The loss of estrogen during this period not only causes dreaded hot flashes, but it can also lead to fatigue, weight gain, and metabolic changes that affect how your body breaks down sugar, potentially resulting in low insulin sensitivity and insulin resistance. That new roll around your middle? Blame it on loss of estrogen, which causes us to lose lean muscle mass and gain abdominal fat.

(See Chapter 7, "Weight, What?") If you experienced anxiety, irritability, panic attacks, brain fog, and migraines during perimenopause, those symptoms may get worse. Women who skated through perimenopause with few symptoms may suddenly find themselves joining their less lucky sisters.

Until you reach that twelve-month mark, the seismic hormonal fluctuations can be confusing and downright frustrating. Consider it the *Am I There Yet?* stage of life. Tracking your symptoms, even if you are unsure if they are due to hormonal fluctuations or external circumstances, can provide you and your doctor with a snapshot of what you're going through.

For Jenny, fifty-three, menopause came as a relief. "The hardest part for me was that my period kept stopping and starting. I would go six months without one and then it would start up again," she says. "I went through three stops and starts over the course of eighteen months. It was exhausting and stressful. My moods were all over the map. I have teenagers and there were times when they would send me over the edge. All the regular problems, like not cleaning their rooms or washing their dishes, were exacerbated. I knew I was overreacting, but I couldn't stop myself. My weight went up and down; I had trouble sleeping, but I chalked it all up to work stress and having to travel a lot for my job. At my annual checkup, my doctor didn't ask about my periods so I didn't bring it up until they finally stopped completely. I was so relieved to be done with it."

That, my friends, is the reset day.

Medically Induced Menopause

Some women have medical conditions that need to be treated in ways that will jump-start menopause early. Menopause can be brought on purposefully through either surgery or medication. Certain cancer treatments can lead to the removal of the ovaries, and chemotherapy or radiation applied to the ovaries can damage them. Some women who suffer from endometriosis and experience painful periods with excessive bleeding opt to have a partial hysterectomy (the uterus is removed but the ovaries are left intact) or a hysterectomy with an oophorectomy (removal of the uterus *and* the ovaries), or choose to use medication (gonadotropin-releasing hormone agonists) that stops menstruation. A hysterectomy with an oophorectomy may offer greater relief from endometrial pain than a hysterectomy alone.

Symptoms start immediately when menopause is medically induced. There is no gradual decline of estrogen and adjusting to symptoms as they ebb and flow. If you know ahead of time that you are due to undergo surgical or medical menopause, speak to your doctor about hormone replacement therapy to alleviate symptoms and lower your disease risk. You can often start within two weeks of a procedure.

One more word about hysterectomies. In the past, most women who underwent this surgery had their ovaries removed at the same time as their uterus. These days, many surgeons try to leave the ovaries intact so that women don't suffer from the abrupt loss of estrogen, although this is not always an option, especially if the reason for the surgery is cancer. It is worth noting that Black women are twice as likely as white women to have their ovaries removed when undergoing hysterectomy, even when there is no discernible medical reason. This is yet another example of the racial disparities in how health care is delivered. Women who have had hysterectomies but still have their ovaries can't get pregnant and will not menstruate, but their ovaries are still producing hormones. They are not officially in menopause, but they may experience an earlier onset than women who did not have surgery. Women who have had their ovaries removed may have an increased risk of heart disease, stroke, cognitive impairment, and loss of libido according to some studies.

The Heat of the Matter: How Long Will It Last?

The loss of estrogen sends your internal cooling system out of whack, and can cause vessels to dilate, leading to increased blood flow that can feel like molten lava rushing through your face, neck, and chest. Officially known as vasomotor symptoms (VMS), hot flashes can be unpredictable and extremely disruptive. One of my patients, Yasmine, compared it to being thrown into a microwave and left to burn from the inside out. Throw in sweating and heart palpitations that can last anywhere from one to five minutes, and follow *that* up with chills, and you can see why hot flashes get such a bad rap.

How hot can it get? Once, when I was out to dinner with my friend Jackie, she began having an intense hot flash. I knew she was going through menopause, but she had never mentioned how bad her symptoms were. Suddenly, while we were waiting for our meal to come, she began having an intense hot flash. Sweat beaded her forehead and she started squirming as she stripped off her sweater. When she ran out of layers to take off, I was convinced that at any moment I was going to see her underwear fly across the room.

Most women's hot flashes start in their face and neck, but Mary, forty-eight, gets zapped with fire in her hands and feet. "I like to say I'm a superhero," she says. "If I put my hands on a wall, they would burn straight through. My husband tells me I should use my hot feet to rub his back like a hot stone massage. As if."

While 80 percent of women experience hot flashes at some point during menopause, certain factors influence when they start, how severe they are, and how long they will last. The earlier you go into perimenopause, the longer you will probably experience hot flashes. (Not fair, I know.) Smoking, drinking alcohol, a high-fat diet, and lack of physical activity can all contribute to turning up the heat. (The good news: these are things you have some control over.) Obesity, high BMI, abdominal fat, and lower socioeconomic status are also linked to more frequent hot flashes.

The Study of Women's Health Across the Nation (SWAN) is considered a hallmark of research into menopause in the U.S., and it highlighted the role race, ethnicity, and life circumstances can play. The study followed women from a variety of backgrounds from the ages of forty-two to fifty-two for over twenty-five years as they transitioned from premenopause through menopause and into early old age.

Japanese American and Chinese American women reported fewer hot flashes and night sweats and less vaginal dryness than Black and white women. Hispanic women reported more urine leakage, vaginal dryness, heart pounding, and forgetfulness than white women. The reasons for these variations are hard to parse. Diet and lifestyle differences among ethnic groups are contributing factors, and symptoms like hot flashes, night sweats, urine leakage, and stiffness or soreness were associated with a high body mass index. Women who were experiencing financial hardship, smoked, or were less physically active than other women their age reported the most symptoms.

There are also racial and ethnic differences in how long symptoms last. The average duration of hot flashes is 4.8 years for Japanese women, 5.4 years for Chinese women, 6.5 years for white women, 8.9 years for Hispanic women, and 10.1 years for Black women.

Life isn't statistics, though, and every woman is different.

Amanda, forty-eight, thought she was prepared for what was to come because both her mother and grandmother went through menopause in their early forties and gave her the low-down. "What they didn't tell me is how intense and frequent hot flashes can be," she says. "They usually start with my face turning bright red. Then my entire body becomes soaked. Sweat will pour down the back of my neck and even my legs. I have terrible body odor. I have to shower four times a day. I even get hot flashes while I'm *in* the shower. If I don't get the cold water running immediately, it feels as if I will have a massive panic attack. I sleep with a fan by my bedside table, another standing fan facing me, and the windows wide open, even in winter. Sometimes my husband gets so cold that he has to go sleep in another room. I can't go anywhere without water, and a one-liter bottle is never enough." Amanda has found that now that she is two years past her last period, the hot flashes are finally beginning to get better. "I'm an outgoing person," she says, "and luckily I was able to talk about it with other women at work, or I would have lost my mind."

Stacy, fifty-one, began getting hot flashes in her late forties. "I started having to dress only in cardigans," she says. "I would get about ten flashes every hour. If I was in the back of a car, I had to roll down all the windows and hang my head out like a dog. I would wake up drenched in the middle of the night and hold my breasts up to keep the sweat from running down my stomach while I ran to the shower." For Stacy, starting hormone replacement therapy made a huge difference. "I may not be ready for turtlenecks yet, but HRT has made it a whole lot better," she says.

The Impact of Hot Flashes on Your Health

Hot flashes aren't just annoying and sometimes, despite our better instincts, embarrassing. They can have a negative impact on sleep, mood, concentration, work, social activities, relationships, and even mortality. Unfortunately, 70 percent of women with moderate to severe hot flashes go untreated, despite viable options, including HRT, that can be hugely beneficial in the short and long term. If I could shout it from the rooftops, I would: *You don't have to suffer this way.* (Hopefully, I'd get a cool breeze while I was up there.)

One of the reasons it's so important to track the frequency and severity of hot flashes and take steps to deal with them is the impact they have on disease risk. In a study of over 11,000 women forty-five to fifty years old, those who experienced frequent hot flashes had an increased risk of developing heart disease, even when the effects of age, menopause status, lifestyle, and other chronic disease risk factors were considered. They are also at higher risk for stroke and high blood pressure. Hot flashes also impact bone health. In a study of over 23,000 postmenopausal women fifty to seventy-nine years old, those with moderate to severe hot flashes had lower bone mineral density and increased rates of hip fractures compared with women who did not have VMS symptoms. Estrogen also plays a critical role in the brain's health and functionality, which is one of the reasons that recent research has linked frequent hot flashes to cognitive decline.

While it may not be appropriate for every patient, hormone replacement therapy (HRT) is the gold standard for treating hot flashes. I'm, admittedly, a big proponent of HRT, but that's because numerous studies have proven its value (and safety) over the years. Don't worry, I'll give you both sides of the story in Chapter 4, "The ABCs of HRT"—in detail!

For now, I will offer you a postscript on my friend Jackie: After she did a striptease in the restaurant, she came into my office and we started her on HRT. Two weeks later, her hot flashes weren't completely gone, but she was no longer tempted to take her clothes off in public.

Diet can also play a role—good and bad—in how you experience hot flashes. Alcohol, caffeine, processed sugar, and high-fat and spicy foods can all be triggers for some women. Because hot flashes are more likely to occur when blood sugar levels dip (like when you skip meals), eating at regular intervals may help slow their frequency.

There is some evidence that eating soy-based products, which are rich in isoflavones, a phytoestrogen that mimics your body's estrogen, can lessen the severity of hot flashes, though it has not proved to be effective with night sweats. Flaxseeds and sesame seeds are other good sources of phytoestrogens.

A diet consisting of mainly lean proteins, whole grains, fruits, vegetables, and olive oil, similar to the Mediterranean diet, which we will talk about in upcoming chapters, may reduce the frequency and severity of hot flashes by up to 20 percent. In addition to including many foods with phytoestrogens, this diet emphasizes eating plenty of nuts and fish. These contain omega-3 fatty acids, which have anti-inflammatory properties and may reduce the severity (though not necessarily the frequency) of hot flashes. There is evidence that women with more fat around their abdomens suffer greater hot flashes, in part because the extra weight acts as heat insulation. Losing weight may help, though there isn't a magic number of pounds proven to do the trick.

There is anecdotal evidence that wild yams and black cohosh, both of which are used in some cultures to treat menopausal symptoms, may help. As I'm sure you can tell by now, I'm a huge believer in food as medicine, but there is not strong research yet to back up these claims. In Chapter 7, we will take a much more extensive look at the role of nutrition in weight loss and health.

Mind Your Hot Flashes

One of the reasons hot flashes can be so disturbing is that you have little control over when they will flare up. Heating up in the middle

---

Did You Know?
How the Severity of Hot Flashes
Is Quantified

While all hot flashes can be miserable, your doctor may ask you to quantify just *how* bad they are. There's a reason. The severity can determine when and if treatment should be started. This is how clinicians define their severity:

- Mild: the sensation of heat without sweating

- Moderate: the sensation of heat with sweating, without the need to discontinue activity

- Severe: the sensation of heat with sweating, causing cessation of activity

---

of giving a presentation at work? On a first date? Arguing with your kids about curfew? There are few (okay, no) good options.

Having a hot flash in public can make you feel as if you are carrying around a giant neon sign announcing, *I am in menopause!* Given the societal stigma, that's pretty much the last thing most women want. I was giving a talk recently when I noticed a woman clinging to the back wall and trying to hide from the audience. Afterward, I went up to her and asked if she was all right. "I could feel a hot flash coming on and I didn't want everyone to see me start sweating," she confessed. Keep in mind, this was at a talk *about* menopause! Let's just say, Generation M is still a work in progress.

You can let yourself feel defeated by your symptoms, but that sense of shame can make an already difficult situation even more upsetting and may even make the hot flashes *themselves* worse. One study that followed over 1,000 women found that having negative beliefs about menopause and, specifically hot flashes, including embarrassment, disgust, feeling out of control, and worrying about how others will react, actually led to more problematic hot flashes. This was particularly true in work situations. Having to speak in public, wear an uncomfortable uniform, or work in a hot and poorly ventilated room added to the stress and precipitated hot flashes.

Instead of letting the mind-body connection work *against* you, there are ways to flip the switch and let it work *for* you. It will take a conscious effort and a bit of work, but it is possible to develop a psychological approach that empowers you to be your biggest cheerleader rather than your harshest critic. Cognitive behavioral therapy (CBT) is a short-term, research-backed form of talk therapy that has proven to be effective at reducing hot flashes by as much as 50 percent and night sweats by 39 percent in menopausal women, regardless of other mitigating factors including age and body weight. It can also lessen depression and improve overall quality of life during menopause in as little as six to ten sessions. (See Chapter 5, "Will I Ever Sleep Again?" for more about how CBT can improve insomnia.)

Unlike other psychotherapies, CBT does not involve delving into your past or resurrecting your childhood. Instead, it focuses on helping you learn better coping skills for your present situation. The goal is to help you interrupt negative thought patterns by identifying distorted beliefs (in this case about menopause) and replace them with

Seven Tips to Turn Down the Heat

These simple lifestyle tips can ease hot flashes when they occur and minimize disruption at work and at night.

1. Dress in layers.

2. Keep an extra blouse or top stashed at work.

3. Put your hair up, or keep a hair tie handy for when a hot flash hits.

4. Carry a cool pack in your bag.

5. Avoid spicy food.

6. Opt for cotton pajamas (and keep an extra pair handy so you don't have to search for them in the night, which risks further disrupting sleep).

7. Switch to bamboo sheets, which tend to stay cooler.

new modes of thinking and behavior that give you a greater sense of control. The first step is to acknowledge your current thought pattern. For example, thinking *I have no control over what my body is doing anymore*, will probably fill you with dread, increase anxiety, and may even make it more likely that a hot flash will occur. You might make a list of these beliefs and next to them write healthier alternatives. For example: *There is nothing shameful about what I am going through.*

Reading through the list every day is one place to start. CBT also teaches stress-reduction techniques, including ways to slow down breathing during tough moments, that can reduce the anxiety, heart palpitations, and fear that make hot flashes worse. The therapy is usually done with a therapist in thirty- to sixty-minute weekly sessions over a period of four to six weeks, in person and via telehealth. There are CBT worksheets online as well.

Coming to terms with aging and changing hormones is definitely a process, but other mind-over-flash methods, including meditation, breath work, and yoga, have also been proven to help. I asked my friend, Dr. Christiane Wolf, a gynecologist *and* meditation teacher, for additional advice on how to deal with the emotional cost of hot flashes. "In mindfulness, there is the concept of primary pain and secondary pain," she told me. "Primary pain is what is actually happening. You are suddenly flushed and sweaty. That is the physical reality. Secondary pain is the negative emotions such as embarrassment, frustration, and fear of loss of control you might have *about* the event: *I will be mortified if I break into a sweat in public.* That secondary pain makes the experience harder and more stressful.

"The first step to developing a more positive mindset is to be cognizant of whether you are adding secondary pain to your situation. When you are in a difficult situation, whether it is caused by a hot flash or a flash of anger, sit for a few minutes and think about what is *actually* happening to you versus how you *feel* about it. Is it making you tense? Depressed? Defeated? Once you become aware of that thought process, you can observe your internal dialog, separate it

BUILDING BLOCK

Learn to STOP

Menopause, with all its symptoms and uncertainties, can be stressful, but there are ways to feel more in control. You've already met my friend the mindfulness expert Dr. Christiane Wolfe. She was kind enough to share one of my favorite techniques to lower anxiety and calm your nervous system. She calls it the STOP practice. I think it's a go.

    S—Stop

    T—Take a breath

    O—Observe what's going on

    P—Proceed

STOP for *awareness*

Use the STOP practice to become fully aware of the present moment: What is going on in the body? The mind? The emotional field? Or ask yourself: "What is *out* of my awareness right now?" It can be as simple as noticing your brain is foggy after being on a conference call for two hours (and that you need a stretch break) or that you have been thinking about the upcoming teacher meeting all morning. Simply stop and take a breath.

STOP for *beauty*

Pause for a moment and notice something beautiful in your surroundings. It can literally be to "stop and smell the roses."

Use all of your senses to find something and then take it in for a breath or two. If that feels too big of a stretch, you can ask yourself: "Okay, I know this is a stressful moment right now, but if there was something beautiful about it, what would it be?" Maybe then we notice the flowers on the table, which blend into the background when we are busy. Or the beautiful braids of the woman in front of us in the (long!) checkout line at the grocery store.

STOP for *compassion*

In a moment of stress or pain, practice STOP to open your heart to kindness and compassion. Compassion is a natural, caring response to suffering, big and small, in ourselves and in others. Sometimes the tug of compassion calls us to stop, at other times we need to stop and really take something in, so we can open the doors of the heart and invite compassion in. Maybe we are a little impatient with our child complaining at length about something that happened at recess. Maybe the adult brain doesn't see it as hurtful, but stopping and truly listening might allow us to connect with the truth of her hurt and allow our heart to melt a little.

from what is physically happening and decide to let go of the secondary pain, or negative self-talk, which is not serving you."

Embarrassment about hot flashes can be particularly pervasive in the workplace. Our society is still steeped in a toxic brew of both sexism and ageism. If you're in a meeting and suddenly have a hot flash, it's easy to feel a sense of fear and assume, *Everyone here thinks I'm too old to be sitting in this chair.* Instead, recognize that your internal dialog stems from insecurity and replace it with the truth, *I'm meant to be sitting in this chair because I have something to offer, including experience, insight, and wisdom.* If nothing else, you can remind yourself that half the time, people are too self-absorbed to even notice.

It may be tempting to write off some of these techniques as too woo-woo, but numerous studies have shown that mindfulness-based and behavioral therapy can help alleviate perimenopausal and menopausal symptoms, including the frequency and intensity of hot flashes, sleep and mood disturbances, depression, stress, and muscle and joint pain, as well as improve overall quality of life. One study of 1,744 women ages forty to sixty-five found that women with higher mindfulness scores had fewer menopausal symptoms, including less irritability and other mood swings. Mindfulness is a broad term that can encompass everything from a two-minute breath-work exercise to a sixty-minute yoga practice. (We'll talk about both.) Essentially, mindfulness simply means bringing awareness to what is going on in your mind and body rather than shifting into an automatic reaction. Once you become aware of your thoughts, you can decide whether or not they serve you, and let them go if not. This can be particularly useful during menopause, when external negativity can compound a body and mind already in flux. The practices can be easily integrated with clinical and other lifestyle approaches. Considering mindfulness is free and safe, and given that you can do it at home, it's at least worth a try.

As menopause becomes more normalized and discussed out in the open, I hope any lingering sense of shame will dissipate. In the meantime, be patient with yourself. One way to have more compassion for yourself is to remember that what you're going through is hard for all women, not just you. That simple acknowledgment can help you release self-blame and start on the path to acceptance. We are truly all in this together.

Lower Your Risk
of These Five Diseases

The loss of estrogen affects your heart, brain, bone, and metabolic health beginning in perimenopause, and the risk increases over the years. The impact is greater for women who experience menopause before age forty-five (considered early menopause) and thus have lower estrogen levels for a longer period of time. A study of 921,517 women who went through early menopause found that they were at higher risk of developing type 2 diabetes, arthritis, sleep apnea, bone fractures, and decreased mobility. They were also at a greater risk of hypertension. Genetics plays a role in all of these diseases, and while you may not have control over your family history, there are modifiable lifestyle factors that you do have a choice about and that can greatly help mitigate the risks.

1. Cardiovascular Disease

Heart disease is the number one killer of women across the world. In part, this is due to the calcifications that begin to form in the blood vessels in both men and women as we get older. For women, a decrease in estrogen compounds these changes. One of estrogen's functions is to keep blood vessels open. When hormone levels decline, a buildup of cholesterol can occur within the arteries, raising the risk of heart disease, high blood pressure, and stroke. It can also result in alterations in your heart rate patterns (how fast or slow your heart beats). Other menopausal symptoms, including sleep disturbances, depression, and weight gain, put additional strain on your heart. Hot flashes and night sweats have also been associated with higher blood pressure and an increased risk of heart disease.

The SWAN study found that the risk of heart disease varies across ethnic and racial groups. Black women experienced more, and earlier, arterial stiffness than white women and, along with Hispanic women, had a higher risk of cardiovascular disease risk in midlife than white and Chinese women.

Perimenopause and menopause are the ideal time to consult with your doctor for a baseline assessment of your cardiovascular health. Screenings can include a stress test, a blood pressure test, and a check of your cholesterol levels. This gives you something to measure against as you begin to take steps to improve your numbers.

In a study of 25,994 women in the U.S., the Mediterranean diet, which emphasizes vegetables, legumes, nuts, and healthy fats, was associated with up to a 28 percent reduction in cardiovascular events. This eating plan lowers biomarkers for inflammation, glucose metabolism, and insulin resistance, and abdominal fat that contributes to heart disease.

Tamar Samuels, a registered dietician who specializes in women's health, has additional nutritional advice for lowering your risk of heart disease. "It's really important to incorporate foods that are high in soluble fiber, such as oats, nuts, apples, and berries," Samuels says. "Soluble fiber acts like a sponge in your system. It soaks up water and helps draw out the cholesterol from food within your gut." A diet high in saturated fat can also lead to an increase in cholesterol, elevated blood sugar, and insulin resistance, which many menopausal women are already prone to because of how estrogen influences insulin production (we'll talk more about this later).

Engaging in physical activity, ideally combining aerobic and strength training exercises, is one of the best ways to improve overall heart health. Stress-reduction techniques, including yoga, meditation, and deep breathing exercises, can all help to lower your blood pressure, as can improving the quantity and quality of your sleep.

We will delve much deeper into HRT, but what you should know for now is that hormone replacement therapy is proven to lower your risk of cardiovascular disease when given before the age of sixty and/or ten years after the last period. (See Chapter 4, "The ABCs of HRT.")

BUILDING BLOCK

Lower Your Risk of Heart Disease

Heart disease remains the number one killer of women, but rather than live in fear, there are proactive steps that can substantially lower your risk, as well as improve your energy and overall quality of life.

- **Exercise.** Regular physical activity can not only strengthen your heart, but also help you maintain a healthy weight. The American Heart Association (AHA) recommends 150 minutes of moderate exercise or 75 minutes of vigorous exercise every week if you are just starting out. Build up from there. (See Chapter 8, "The Exercise Rx.")

- **A diet that includes fruits, vegetables, nuts,** and limited processed food can lower your risk of heart disease. The Mediterranean diet, which includes fruits, vegetables, nuts, and olive oil and limits the amount of red meat and dairy, has been shown to lower the risk of heart disease and reduce cholesterol, according to the AHA.

- **Lower your salt intake.** Diets high in sodium result in a 19 percent increase in heart disease. Skip the table salt and limit processed foods that tend to be high in sodium.

- **Prioritize sleep.** Ongoing and long-term loss of sleep can increase the risk of hypertension, high blood pressure, and cardiovascular disease. (See Chapter 5, "Will I Ever Sleep Again?" for strategies to get a better night's sleep.)

- **Reduce stress.** Slowing down your rate of inhalations and exhalations can reduce your heart rate, lower the risk of hypertension, and decrease stress and inflammatory responses. Try this simple "square breathing" technique whenever you are feeling stressed: Inhale to the count of four, hold for the count of four, exhale to the count of four. Repeat two to three times or until you feel calmer.

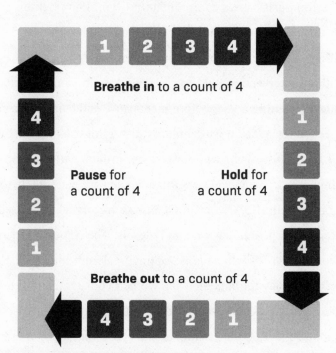

Breathe in to a count of 4

Pause for a count of 4

Hold for a count of 4

Breathe out to a count of 4

2. Osteoporosis

The loss of estrogen decreases calcium absorption and is the most common cause of osteoporosis, a weakening of bone density and deterioration of bone tissue. The biggest risk associated with osteoporosis is bone fractures. The Centers for Disease Control (CDC) found that one in four Americans over the age of sixty-five will fall, which is the leading cause of fatal and nonfatal injuries among older adults. For women with osteoporosis, the risk of a fall that leads to a life-altering fracture is even higher. An estimated 50 percent of women over fifty years old will experience an osteoporosis-related fracture, often with devastating consequences in terms of disability, mortality, and personal costs. Society at large pays a cost as well. Osteoporosis causes approximately 1.9 million fractures every year in the United States, at an estimated annual health-care cost of $57 billion. Falling once doubles the risk of falling again.

Without intervention, the rate of bone loss in women increases dramatically starting a year before menopause and persists for up to three years after. Women with a family history of osteoporosis, with a small body frame, and who have gone through early menopause are at higher risk. Asian and Caucasian women are more likely to get osteoporosis than Black women. Other risk factors include a sedentary life, smoking, and low vitamin D levels. The National Osteoporosis Foundation recommends an optimal calcium intake of 1,000 milligrams per day for both men and women younger than fifty, with an increase to 1,200 milligrams for those fifty and older. It also recommends 800 to 1,000 international units (IU) per day of vitamin D for men and women over fifty.

A bone density test (DEXA scan) is a painless, noninvasive test that can measure your degree of bone loss and is often recommended for all women at age sixty-five. This can help your doctor determine what steps you can take, including medications that can prevent osteoporosis from worsening and in some cases can even help rebuild bone. There are a number of options, including daily and monthly pills, and infusions, depending on your personal health status.

The most common medications are bisphosphonates (for example, Boniva and Fosamax). These are generally the first-line treatment for osteoporosis and are quite effective, but bisphosphonates can have side effects. The most serious, though rare, complication is osteonecrosis (bone deterioration) of the jaw. If you take bisphosphonates, let your dentist or oral surgeon know before any procedure. Some patients also report gastrointestinal effects, such as acid reflux and esophageal irritation.

Because DEXA scans are not usually covered by insurance until a woman is sixty-five, osteoporosis often goes undiagnosed until then. That's one of the reasons I feel so strongly about the importance of taking *preventive* steps in your forties and fifties. One of the most effective is estrogen replacement therapy, which has been shown to reduce osteoporosis-related fractures by approximately 50 percent when started soon after menopause and continued long term.

Priya Patel is the founder of Wellen, an exercise program designed specifically for women at risk for osteoporosis. "One of the biggest problems I see today is that younger women are not thinking about bone health," she says. "They are not aware of what they should be doing to improve bone density until they are already diagnosed with osteoporosis. That's unfortunate because this is the best time to make a difference."

Fall prevention comes down to three main components: balance, strength, and posture. We will dive much deeper into specific exercises and their benefits in Chapter 8, "The Exercise Rx," but I asked Patel to talk a little bit more about posture, which is often overlooked. "Posture is especially important for women at risk of osteoporosis to prevent vertebral compression of the spine, which can leave you permanently hunched and at a greater risk for falls," she says. "Most women think about strengthening their core to improve posture. That's great, but it's not everything. It's just as important to strengthen your upper arm and back muscles to maintain good alignment *before* you hit menopause. This is an area, too, where most women are particularly weak."

Here's a quick test to see where (and how!) you stand: Stand against a wall in your normal position. If your full body is not in contact with the wall, chances are you need to work on your posture. To improve your posture, practice pushing your shoulders and upper back up against the wall. This will help activate the muscles that need strengthening.

Hip fractures are a particularly devastating result of osteoporosis. Along with working on your posture, improving the strength of your glute (i.e., butt!) and thigh muscles can protect your hip bones. A simple "bridge" exercise is a good place to start. Lie on your back with your knees bent and your feet planted on the floor an arm's length away from your butt. Keeping the rest of your body planted, slowly lift your hips up off the ground. Hold for a count of five, then lower down. Repeat this ten times, being mindful not to arch your back.

Some loss of balance is a natural occurrence with aging, but it doesn't have to be inevitable. Practicing tai chi not only lowers blood pressure and calms the mind, the slow, circular movements involved are also proven to improve balance and can reduce falls by up to 50 percent. A few quick home exercises incorporating both dynamic (moving) and static (say, standing still on one leg) movements can improve your balance in just six weeks. A dynamic exercise you can do while going about your life (cooking, taking a break from your desk) is simply marching slowly in place.

One of my go-to fitness experts is Hailey Babcock, who specializes in training women over forty. She recommends doing this two-minute practice every day.

- Stand on one leg and slowly raise the other leg with your knee bent. If you are unsteady, rest your hands on a table or top of chair until you can hold the pose for sixty seconds. Switch legs and repeat.

- Once you are secure with this, stand on one leg with the other knee bent and pass a light weight (even a can will do) back and forth between your hands while balancing. Repeat on the other leg.

One activity that truly stands out for bone health and fall prevention is yoga. Just twelve minutes of yoga a day can improve bone mineral density in your spine, hips, and femur. Better yet, it improves

What to Eat for Stronger Bones

Calcium, protein, and vitamin D are all important to protect against osteoporosis. While vitamin D comes from sunshine, it can sometimes be hard to get enough in your diet without supplementation. Your doctor can measure your vitamin D levels and discuss whether calcium and magnesium supplements can help you with bone health. The standard recommendation is to aim for 1,000 to 1,200 milligrams of calcium a day, along with protein, to help build and protect bones. The Cleveland Clinic suggests these sources:

- **Dairy products** have the highest calcium content. Dairy products include milk, yogurt, and cheese. A cup (8 ounces) of milk contains 300 milligrams of calcium. The calcium content is the same for skim, low fat, and whole milk.

- **Fruits and dark green, leafy vegetables** contain high amounts of calcium, vitamin K, folate, magnesium, and potassium, as well as antioxidants such as vitamin C and carotenoids, which are associated with greater bone mineral density.

- **Canned salmon or sardines** both have about 200 milligrams of calcium and are good additions to a green salad.

- **Cereal, pasta, breads, and other food** made with whole grains that are fortified with minerals, including folate and calcium.

posture, balance, and coordination. And it leads to greater range of motion, more strength, and less anxiety. (See Chapter 8, "The Exercise Rx," for more on different types of yoga and tai chi.)

As with any exercise, be sure to check with your doctor first. If you have osteoporosis, tell your yoga instructor at the beginning of class. You may be instructed to avoid anything that involves twisting your spine. There are a number of yoga classes specifically designed for osteoporosis on YouTube and other online platforms.

3. Thyroid Disease

The thyroid is a small, butterfly-shaped gland in the front of your neck. It produces hormones that play a crucial role in regulating metabolic function, including body temperature, energy expenditure, and heart rate. These hormones include triiodothyronine (T3) and thyroxine (T4). Because the thyroid is affected by estrogen levels, women are more likely to develop thyroid disease than men. Other factors that play a role include genetics, stress, environmental factors, autoimmune diseases, and aging.

Women are more likely to develop an underactive thyroid, *hypothyroidism*, during menopause than an overactive thyroid, *hyperthyroidism*. In fact, up to 20 percent of menopausal and postmenopausal women suffer from hypothyroidism. The symptoms can mimic those associated with menopause, including hot flashes, loss of libido, weight gain, fatigue, insomnia, and heart palpitations. Some research suggests that an underactive thyroid can make menopausal symptoms worse. Symptoms of hyperthyroidism include anxiety, tremors, and difficulty sleeping.

Changes in the Body with Thyroid Abnormalities

Brain/CNS
Impaired mentation
Impaired memory
Confusion
Altered mood
Depression

Facial Features
Periorbital edema
Loss of hair

Voice Changes
Hoarseness

Goiter
Dysphagia

Breast
Impaired lactation

Respiratory System
Decreased respiratory
   drive
Hypercapnia
Hypoxemia

Liver
Cholesterol regulation
Increased total cholesterol
Increased LDL cholesterol
Increased lipoprotein A
Decreased hepatic proteins
   (e.g., SHBG)
Decreased gluconeogenesis

Renal
Reduced GFR
Hyponatremia
Urinary retention

Muscle
Weakness
Muscle fatigability
Cramping and stiffness
Decreased glucose
   uptake

Skin and Nails
Dry skin
Cool skin
Edematous skin
Brittle nails

Gastrointestinal System
Constipation
Decreased motility
Increased edema
Decreased bowel sounds
Abdominal distention

Hematological System
Impaired immune response
Impaired coagulation
Anemia

THE MAIN EVENT AND THE AFTER-PARTY

Temperature Regulation
Cold intolerance
Altered energy partitioning
Regulation of SNS effects on
  fat, muscle, and liver

CNS: Central Nervous System

SNS: Sympathetic Nervous System

SHBG: Sex Hormone Binding Globulin

BAT: Brown Adipose Tissue

WAT: White Adipose Tissue

Pituitary
Elevated TSH levels

Hair
Thinning hair
Hair loss
Alopecia

Heart, Cardiac System
Reduced heart rate
Bradycardia
Impaired systolic function
Impaired diastolic function
Increased systolic time intervals
Impaired contractility
Pericardial effusion

Adipose tissue
Decreased thermogenesis (BAT)
Decreased lipolysis (WAT)

Reproductive System
Infertility
Menstrual irregularities
Menometrorrhagia

Examples of Multi-Organ Effects
Fatigue
Decreased basal metabolic rate
Decreased exercise intolerance
Weight gain
Increased body mass index

Bone
Decreased bone turnover
Reduced bone resorption
Decreased bone formation

Peripheral Nervous System
Diminished reflexes
Delayed Achilles and patellar reflexes

Despite how common it is, thyroid disease often goes undiagnosed because the symptoms can overlap with those caused by menopause and the aging process itself. Left untreated, though, thyroid disease can lead to an increased risk of heart disease, bone fractures, cognitive impairment, and depression. A simple blood test can measure the levels of T3, T4, and two other thyroid-related hormones (TRH and TSH) to determine if you have thyroid disease. If you do, it can be treated with medication, with a targeted dosage determined by your blood test results in conjunction with how well your symptoms are being managed.

When thyroid medications were first developed, they were made from animal sources, including the thyroid glands of pigs or cows. Today, first-line treatment is usually monotherapy with levothyroxine, a synthetic form of T4 that your body converts to T3 and that is designed to mimic these hormones. It is FDA-approved and available from several pharmaceutical manufacturers. One of the most common brand names is Synthroid.

Every person converts T4 to T3 at different rates, and monotherapy may not address those differences. Combination therapy in the form of desiccated thyroid extract made from animal thyroid glands is available as Armour® Thyroid and Nature-Throid®. While these are not FDA-approved, they may be suitable for women who are not getting the desired results from synthetics or prefer a more natural alternative.

As an added bonus, thyroid medications may also help menopausal symptoms and can be taken with HRT. When you first start thyroid medication, your doctor will probably do blood tests every six to eight weeks to see how your body is responding and tweak the dosage accordingly. After that, once or twice a year usually suffices to check levels for as long as you are on the medication. Many people remain on medication for the rest of their lives.

One of the most common forms of hypothyroidism is Hashimoto's thyroiditis, an autoimmune disease that causes your immune system to attack your thyroid. Women are seven to ten times as likely to get Hashimoto's as men, probably due to fluctuating hormone levels. It tends to first occur when you are thirty to fifty years old. White Americans are twice as likely to be diagnosed with Hashimoto's disease compared to people who are Black, Asian, and Pacific Islanders. Hispanic people experience Hashimoto's disease at higher rates than people who are Black, Asian, and Pacific Islander, but not as high as people who are white. Like other forms of hypothyroidism, Hashimoto's is treated by supplementing with T3 and/or T4 hormones.

While there is no perfect thyroid level for all women, it is possible for blood tests to show that your levels are in the "normal" range and still have a thyroid that is not functioning at optimal level. Symptoms include unexplained fatigue, weight gain, thinning eyebrows, and brittle hair.

Nutrition plays a big role, whether or not you have been diagnosed with thyroid disease. "Iron helps your thyroid to function," Tamar Samuels explains. "Good sources include red meat, shellfish, beans, and spinach. Selenium is another essential mineral that acts as an antioxidant and is important for a healthy thyroid. You can meet your needs for selenium with just one Brazil nut a day. Iodine is also essential. Most of us get enough from traditional iodized table salt, and seafood, eggs, and seaweed are also good sources of iodine." Samuels doesn't recommend iodine supplements, which can cause symptoms to flare up.

For women with Hashimoto's, Samuels recommends an anti-inflammatory eating plan. Our good friend, the Mediterranean diet, is one to keep in mind. "Olive oil, avocado oil, and nuts all have omega-three fatty acids, which are particularly powerful when it comes to combating inflammation," she says. "Fatty fish like salmon, mackerel, and tuna are all good sources of omega-threes, as are walnuts, flax seeds and chia seeds."

4. Metabolic Syndrome

There are estrogen receptors all over your body that help to regulate insulin, the hormone produced in your pancreas that regulates glucose (sugar) in the bloodstream. One of insulin's primary functions is to facilitate the uptake of glucose by cells, including muscle cells, which need it for fuel. When estrogen levels decline, your sensitivity to insulin decreases, too, which can throw your pancreas into overdrive and leave too much sugar in your bloodstream because your muscles and other cells aren't properly absorbing it. This inability to utilize sugar efficiently can result in insulin resistance. If you've ever wondered why a single glass of wine hits you harder as you go through perimenopause and menopause, it's because when estrogen levels are low, you can't process the sugar in alcohol as effectively. And yes, this can also result in weight gain.

Insulin resistance raises the risk of metabolic syndrome, a cluster of risk factors for cardiovascular disease, inflammation, high blood pressure, and type 2 diabetes. Changes in body composition common in menopause, including a decrease in lean muscle mass and an increase in abdominal (visceral fat), can make this even more likely. Women who have gone through surgically induced menopause, with its abrupt cessation of estrogen, are at higher risk of developing insulin resistance and metabolic syndrome.

HRT can significantly reduce the risk of metabolic syndrome and diabetes, especially when it is started early in menopause. Strength training and eating a healthy, low-sugar diet can also help you build and maintain the lean muscle you need to offset insulin resistance.

"When insulin resistance is not well-controlled, either with diet, lifestyle, and/or medication, it can become a vicious cycle," Tamar Samuel says. "When blood sugar is low, you tend to crave highly processed carbohydrates. This type of food goes through your system very quickly and causes a spike in blood sugar. Your pancreas will have to work extra hard to get that blood sugar down by pumping out a lot of insulin."

One way to interrupt this cycle is to be sure to eat protein with carbohydrates. "Protein takes longer to digest and slows that process down, resulting in a more gradual release of glucose into the bloodstream," Samuels says. "It also helps you to stay full longer, which can help with weight loss." Eating meals at regular times can help keep your blood sugar levels even.

A short walk can help your body absorb glucose from your bloodstream into your cells, where it's converted and utilized for fuel. Finally, managing stress also helps. That's because during the fight-or-flight response, cortisol and blood sugar increase, which can end up making you more insulin resistant. Exercise, meditation, yoga, and breath work (yes, I'm mentioning them again) can help manage stress and positively impact metabolic syndrome.

5. Bladder Health

Estrogen loss during menopause can cause changes to the vulva, urethra, and bladder, and can also make the vaginal walls thinner, drier, and inflamed. These symptoms are part of what's now called the genitourinary syndrome of menopause (GSM), which includes genital, sexual, and urinary symptoms related to changes that happen during menopause. (We'll talk more about the impact on sex in upcoming chapters.)

There are estrogen receptors in the bladder and throughout the lower urinary tract. Declining estrogen levels can result in a thinning of the lining of the urethra (the short tube that passes urine from the bladder), a decreased ability for the urinary sphincter to contract, and a reduced ability for the bladder to hold large amounts of urine.

This can lead to incontinence, as well as an overactive bladder, which makes you feel like you need to pee more frequently, especially during the night. Symptoms include urine leakage when you laugh, sneeze, cough, jump, or lift heavy objects, and they usually begin during perimenopause.

Urinary tract infections (UTIs) become more common during menopause because the loss of estrogen lowers the vaginal pH, which reduces the acidity that helps fight "bad" bacteria, yeast, and infection. At the same time, it decreases the amount of "good" bacteria, lactobacillus, which is the dominant vaginal flora in premenopausal women and plays a crucial role in preventing the overgrowth of harmful microorganisms. Symptoms include burning, the frequent need to pee, cloudy or strong-smelling urine, pelvic pressure, and/or blood in the urine. These can be treated by antibiotics if necessary.

It's important to report any symptoms to your doctor. Thirty-three million Americans are dealing with an overactive bladder, thirteen million have urinary incontinence, and 81,000 are diagnosed with bladder cancer each year. If you experience any changes in your urinary habits, see blood in your urine, or are experiencing leakage, talk to your doctor to rule out non-menopausal causes.

Don't wait until bladder issues get so severe that they impact your quality of life, including your ability to exercise, get a good night's sleep, and participate in your social life, due to fear of incontinence. Early intervention with lifestyle changes and medication, if necessary, can make a big difference. Topical estrogen therapy in the form of tablets or creams can relieve urinary symptoms, including frequency and urgency, and can reduce the likelihood of recurrent UTIs in postmenopausal women. If you are experiencing burning when you pee, your diet may also be a contributing factor. Triggers are highly personal, but common irritants include acidic foods, citrus, caffeine, and carbonated beverages.

Other "down there" issues also become more common during menopause. Estrogen receptors have been identified in all major structural components that provide support to pelvic organs, including the ligaments that connect your uterus to the base of your spine, the vagina, and pelvic floor muscles. Loss of estrogen can cause pelvic floor muscles to weaken, much like other muscles in your body. This can lead to prolapse, when your pelvis, bladder, bowel, and uterus drop, resulting in further loss of control. Menopausal weight gain can exacerbate this. Symptoms include a sensation of vaginal bulge and increased vaginal pressure or heaviness. Pelvic prolapse can be diagnosed by a doctor through pelvic strength and bladder function tests, an MRI, and/or an ultrasound. Estrogen treatment can help, as can exercises to strengthen the pelvis. Remember Kegels? It's time to bring them back. Depending on the severity, minimally invasive surgery can help by securing the tissue between the rectum and vagina and, if necessary, reducing extra tissue.

CHAPTER FOUR

The ABCs of HRT

The art of decision-making includes the art of questioning.

—PEARL ZHU

The theory behind hormone replacement therapy (HRT) sounds relatively clear-cut: replace the hormones that decrease during menopause with synthetic or natural equivalents to ease symptoms and reduce long-term disease risk.

Of course, it is nowhere near that clear-cut in practice. Quite the opposite.

When it comes to menopause there is no topic as controversial, confusing, and at times, concerning to women as HRT.

Before I go into the history, pros, and cons, I want to be totally transparent about where I'm coming from. I believe that for most women HRT can be safe and can have a transformative effect on how you experience menopause. It can not only reduce or alleviate symptoms, from hot flashes to vaginal dryness, it can also help to protect against heart disease, certain cancers, osteoporosis, and diabetes. It has the potential to lower your overall risk of mortality and increase your health span (the number of years you live enjoying good health). Something harder to quantify but equally important: HRT can bring back a sense of vitality at a time of life when many women are faced with a range of emotional challenges brought on by hormonal shifts.

That said, HRT is not appropriate for all women at all times, and it must always be considered carefully with your doctor in light of your personal medical history. My goal is to ensure that you make an informed decision based on the latest facts from a full range of scientifically validated research.

One of the things that frustrates me is the number of women I meet who could have been helped by HRT but never even considered it due to fear based on a single study done by the Women's Health Initiative (WHI) over two decades ago. (It's worth repeating. We're talking about one study done over twenty years ago.) This study showed that using estrogen plus progestin hormone replacement therapy raised the risk of heart disease, stroke, blood clots, breast cancer, and dementia, so it rightly scared a lot of people. However, in the years that followed, the WHI study was shown to have been deeply flawed. The average age of participants was sixty-three years (well past the onset of menopause for most women) and went all the way up to age seventy-nine, so, as a group, they were more at risk

GINNI'S STORY

I was worried about the risks at first.

At my last checkup my doctor asked how long it was since my last period, and I wasn't entirely sure. She took the initiative and probed about my symptoms. I told her I was having trouble sleeping. I wasn't my usual optimistic self. I felt flat but I couldn't put my finger on it. I'm glad she asked, because until then, I didn't associate what I was going through with hormonal changes. I was reticent when she bought up HRT because I had heard so much about the risks involved that I hadn't really considered it. My doctor explained that there had been a lot of misleading information that came out in the late nineties. She outlined all the reasons that she thought that it was safe and probably valuable for me to start now rather than waiting. She assured me that I would be getting regular mammograms and all the health checks necessary. I went home and thought about it for a month before deciding that, for me, there were more upsides than risks. Once I started, my hot flashes stopped within a month and I started sleeping again. Emotionally, it felt like a cloud had lifted. The only thing I don't like about the patch is that it leaves a sticky adhesive on my belly, but that's a small price to pay.

—Ginni, 51

for metabolic disorders, cancer, and dementia, regardless of any hormone therapy. The combination therapy (estrogen plus progestin) did show a modest increase in risk for breast cancer, but only after five years of continuous use. (And after twenty years, their risk of mortality matched that of the control group, further negating these effects.) The hormones in the WHI study were given at higher doses and different formulations than the ones prescribed today. Later research not only discounted many of its original findings but concluded that in most cases, the benefits of HRT, including the prevention of a number of diseases that affect quality of life and longevity, like heart disease and osteoporosis, outweigh the potential risks for most women. Nevertheless, it is taking a while for that message to get through.

Linda, fifty-six, went into menopause ten years ago. She suffered from painful sex, mood swings, and insomnia but her doctor never brought up the possibility of HRT, and she didn't ask about it. "I remembered reading that HRT could cause cancer and that terrified me, even though my symptoms were making me miserable," she says. "Just thinking about taking hormones sent me into a panic. Three years ago, when I had basically stopped sleeping, I went to a new doctor who explained to me that the latest research about HRT showed that my personal risk is actually quite low, so I decided to give it a try," Linda says. "The difference it has made to my life is enormous. I'm finally able to really enjoy myself, and my sex life, again. I'm angry that I lost out on some good years unnecessarily because I didn't have a complete picture of the facts."

When it comes to HRT, as in all things in life, knowledge is power. Knowledge about the latest research and the newest treatment options. Knowledge about your own disease risk factors. Knowledge, too, that you are entitled to take all the time you need and ask all the questions you want, and you can always change your mind. Information, personalization, and self-determination are the core tenets of Generation M.

It's worth the time to take a closer look at the root of so many of the concerns about HRT. Most of the anxiety stems from the WHI study that was conducted from the 1990s to the early 2000s and has since proved to be far less than perfect in its construct, cohort, and conclusions.

The original goal of the research, which followed 27,347 women ages fifty to seventy-nine, was to explore whether hormone replacement treatment could reduce the risk of heart disease and mortality. A secondary goal was to examine the effect on bone fractures and determine whether breast cancer was a potential risk. The study was never intended to examine the effects of HRT on menopausal symptoms including hot flashes, insomnia, and vaginal dryness, all of which decrease quality of life and can increase the risk of a range of diseases. The average age of participants was sixty-three. That's more than ten years older than when we now recommend starting HRT. The majority had already gone through menopause. That fact alone puts the relevance of the research under question for menopausal women.

But here's what happened. Five years into the WHI study, researchers found an increased risk of breast cancer, stroke, pulmonary embolism, and myocardial infarction in women taking combined estrogen and progestin, although it found lower incidence of fracture due to osteoporosis. On May 31, 2002, the WHI prematurely halted the study. The results were widely publicized, and the use of HRT plunged off a cliff. What was not widely publicized at the time was that the trial was riddled with problems that led to misleading conclusions and scared women unnecessarily.

These problems include the age of the participants chosen, the types of hormones used, and the fact that researchers did not take the women's previous risk factors into account.

Let's look at heart disease first. The average age of the women in the study was sixty-three; one-third of the participants had hypertension and one-half had a history of smoking, all of which put them at increased risk for cardiac disease. Many were already receiving medication for hypertension. Only 10 percent of the women in the study were at an age when HRT might have proven to be effective against the development and progression of heart disease. Further studies have shown that hormone therapy can significantly reduce the risk of cardiac disease when given to women fifty to fifty-nine years old (the current recommendation).

The biggest news flash from the study that led to the most pervasive fear was the report of a heightened risk of breast cancer. Here, too, the results were overstated and based on questionable methodology. There was no examination of the role different doses or the types of estrogen or progesterone used might play. Participants were not screened for preexisting risk factors for breast cancer, including obesity and family history. Plus, the study used only one type of synthetic progesterone, progestin. Many forms of progesterone we use today have a lower risk profile for breast cancer.

The women in the WHI study were divided into three groups. Women with a uterus were given estrogen and progestin. Women without a uterus were given estrogen alone. The third group was given a placebo. The women who were given estrogen alone did not show an increase in breast cancer, though the women given estrogen with progestin did experience an increased incidence of the disease. Even that increase was the equivalent of the (slightly) heightened risk from drinking two glasses of wine a day. Still, when it came to publicity, the results focused only on the group given estrogen and progestin, and the risk, I believe, was blown out of proportion.

To recap: We have a study based on a majority of women older than we now recommend HRT for, many of whom had preexisting risk factors for disease and who were given a hormone that is no longer in wide use.

Whether HRT increases the risk of breast cancer, and if so, by how much, has been widely researched since then. Most studies published since 2000 show that estrogen alone does not increase the risk of breast cancer, or if it does, only to a very small degree. The American Cancer Society has stated that in its view taking estrogen alone does not increase the risk of breast cancer, but it might raise the risk of endometrial cancer in women with a uterus. It has been found that the risk of breast cancer rises the longer you stay on HRT, which is why it is usually recommended to stop after five years. Once you stop taking HRT, your risk of breast cancer gradually declines. Keep in mind, though, that there may be reasons for some women to stay on

HRT longer, especially if their risk is higher for other conditions, say heart disease, than breast cancer.

Recent research has shown that the benefits of HRT outweigh the risks for most women. The North American Menopause Society (NAMS) concluded, "Hormone therapy is the most effective treatment for hot flashes and vaginal dryness associated with menopause as well as the prevention of bone loss and fracture, although risks depend on type, dose, duration of use, route of administration, and timing of initiation." It went on to say, "The benefits of hormone therapy outweigh the risks for most healthy symptomatic women who are younger than sixty years and within ten years of menopause onset." For women who have gone through premature or early menopause (before the age of forty-five), and are thus at higher risk of bone loss, heart disease, and cognitive or mood disorders, NAMS states that hormone therapy can be used until at least the average age of menopause (approximately fifty-one), unless there is a contraindication.

Nevertheless, the WHI ripple effect is still being felt all these years later, despite these findings. Sarah, forty-three, had a hysterectomy four years ago and immediately went into menopause. "I had night sweats, hot flashes, and such bad brain fog I could barely remember a thing. I was snapping at my kids and just generally miserable. In retrospect, it seems crazy that my surgeon didn't bring up the potential of starting HRT. It was only when I went to see a menopause specialist that they recommended hormones. I had all my blood work done and ended up getting estrogen as well as progesterone to help me sleep. It turned

BUILDING BLOCK

Five Things to Remember
When Talking to Your Doctor About HRT

I suggest you make a separate appointment with a doctor well-versed in the topic to talk about HRT so that you have time to go over all your options along with your personal medical history. Because it's easy to forget the questions you meant to ask, bring this list with you. Ask your doctor if they are okay with you recording the conversation so that you can go over the details later as you consider your options.

1. **Review your personal disease risk profile and family history,** including diabetes, heart disease, osteoporosis, cholesterol levels, breast cancer, blood clots, and colon cancer.

2. **Discuss which symptoms are most impacting your quality of life,** including hot flashes, vaginal dryness, sleep disorders, and mood disorders, as this may affect which HRT is best for you.

3. **Ask for a full explanation of the types of HRT available,** including pharmaceutical and bioidentical options.

4. **Consider your lifestyle preferences,** including whether a daily pill is right for you or a longer-lasting, less frequently delivered option.

5. **List all supplements,** herbs, vitamins, and current medications you are using. Certain supplements, including St. John's wort, ginkgo biloba, and melatonin, may interfere with how HRT is absorbed.

out I also needed thyroid medication. Now, I have more energy. I'm sleeping better and my mood has improved. The combination of all three has really changed my life. I wish I had been more proactive sooner and asked more questions about my symptoms."

Piraye Yurttas Beim, PhD, is founder of Celmatix Inc., a preclinical-stage women's health biotech focused uniquely on ovarian biology. A renowned expert on the role of hormones, she has this to say: "A lot of research that's come out in recent years shows that for most women, HRT not only helps manage their menopausal symptoms, making their experience more comfortable, but it may fundamentally impact their longevity and overall wellness. Estrogen and ovarian hormones, including progesterone, which is typically part of the HRT formulation, are vital for many functions throughout the body, including mental health, bone health, cardiovascular and immune function, and metabolism. The loss of ovarian function is the single biggest accelerant of unhealthy aging in women," Dr. Beim says. "HRT is not the fountain of youth, but it can play a big role in helping you age in the healthiest possible way through your seventies, eighties and beyond."

HRT and Racial Disparities

Unfortunately, as with so much in health care, there are racial disparities in how HRT is administered in the treatment of menopause. A 2022 report in *Menopause, The Journal of The Menopause Society* disclosed the persistence of this insipid problem.

The study "Racial/Ethnic Disparities in the Diagnosis and Management of Menopause Symptoms among Midlife Women Veterans" was conducted by the Veterans Administration and followed 200,901 women. The research showed that despite Black women veterans experiencing more burdensome menopausal symptoms, they were less likely to get hormone therapy than white participants. The type of HRT prescribed also differed according to ethnicity. Hispanic/Latinx women veterans were less likely to be prescribed systemic HRT and more likely to be prescribed vaginal estrogen alone, regardless of what symptoms they were experiencing. While that is an appropriate choice for many women, the type of HRT women receive should be tailored to their specific symptoms and medical history, not their ethnicity.

We have to do better than this.

So, What Exactly Is in HRT?

HRT can contain a mix of hormones (usually estrogen and progesterone) or a single hormone (usually estrogen). Testosterone is sometimes included. Before we get into different formulations and delivery systems, let's take a look at the role each of these hormones plays in HRT.

Estrogen

Most estrogen is produced in the ovaries, though some also comes from the adrenal glands, fat tissue, brain, breasts, liver, and muscles.

There are estrogen receptors (i.e., the protein in cells that kicks estrogen into action) throughout your body, including in your gut, brain, bones, liver, colon, and even your skin and hair. That's why virtually every organ is affected when estrogen levels begin to dip during perimenopause and menopause. Estrogen also serves to regulate your body's temperature.

There are three main types of estrogen that play different roles: estrone (E1) is a weaker form of estrogen usually found in postmenopause; estradiol (E2) is the predominant form of estrogen in women, especially during their reproductive years; and estriol (E3) helps prepare the uterus to give birth. As women go from early perimenopause to late menopause, levels of estradiol (E2) begin to decline significantly, causing symptoms from night sweats to metabolic disorders and panic attacks. (We'll get into each of these.)

Supplemental estrogen not only alleviates hot flashes and vaginal dryness, it can also protect against heart disease, inflammation, bone-weakening, and fractures due to osteoporosis. It may protect against muscle damage and even speed muscle repair. In fact, one study showed that postmenopausal women on estrogen hormone therapy had greater physical strength than those without treatment.

Progesterone

Progesterone works with estrogen to enhance mood and sleep by regulating receptors in the brain. It helps to quell anxiety, regulate blood pressure, and control the bladder. Progesterone also helps build bones, improves visual memory, and has a beneficial effect on the immune system. Because progesterone protects the lining of the uterus, it is combined with estrogen to lower the risk of endometrial cancer for women who have not had a hysterectomy. HRT can use different doses and types of progesterone, including synthetic or bioidentical. (Don't worry, I'm going to do a deep dive into the difference.) Some studies have found the progesterone used in bioidentical hormones has a lower risk of causing breast cancer than the synthetic hormones used in pharmaceutical HRT. One additional thing to note: some forms of HRT can also cause the return of monthly bleeding that is similar to your previous periods, so don't be alarmed if you see this once you start therapy.

Testosterone

We tend to think of testosterone as a strictly male hormone, but women have testosterone receptors in almost all tissues, including the breasts, heart, blood vessels, gastrointestinal tract, brain, and bladder. When testosterone levels drop during menopause, it can have a detrimental effect on energy levels, libido, and mood, and can lead to loss of lean muscle mass. Supplemental testosterone may improve sex drive, energy, and overall well-being. Standard pharmaceutical HRT does not include testosterone, though it can be prescribed separately, and is currently not FDA approved for women. Doctors may include testosterone in the formula of compounded bioidentical hormones. Stay tuned for more on that.

Know Your Personal Risk Factors

When making a decision whether or not to use HRT, and which hormones might be most appropriate for you, it is important to take your personal risk factors for specific diseases into account.

Breast cancer: Lifestyle factors that increase the likelihood of breast cancer include a sedentary lifestyle, smoking, drinking, and obesity. You can address these risk factors, but there are others that you can't control, including having dense breasts, a family history of breast cancer, radiation to the breasts at an early age, genetic predisposition, and having your first child after the age of thirty-five. Some evidence suggests HRT doesn't increase the risk of breast cancer in women with the BRCA 1 or 2 genes, but it should be carefully considered with your doctor. Systemic HRT is generally not advised for breast cancer survivors, but even here the thinking continues to evolve. A recent influential study in *JAMA* (*Journal of American Medical Association*) suggests that topical vaginal estrogen may be safe for breast cancer survivors, with no increase in mortality. All women, regardless of whether they use HRT and what type, should be diligent about getting regular mammograms.

Ovarian cancer: This is the deadliest reproductive system cancer and the fifth leading cause of cancer-related deaths in women in the United States. Certain lifestyle factors actually decrease the risk of ovarian cancer, including breastfeeding, use of oral contraceptives, and multiple pregnancies. Factors that increase the risk include obesity, diabetes, miscarriages, and a family history of breast or ovarian cancer. Data regarding the effects of HRT on ovarian cancer is often contradictory, but most studies show that HRT that contains both estrogen and progesterone can increase the risk, especially when given to women over fifty years old. When women under fifty were given estrogen alone, there did not appear to be an increased risk.

Endometrial cancer: A high fat diet, obesity, and a sedentary lifestyle increase your risk of endometrial cancer. It is also twice as likely to occur in women with type 2 diabetes. That doesn't rule out HRT, but it does make the choice of what type extremely important. Endometrial cancer thrives on exposure to estrogen. On the other hand, progesterone helps to protect against endometrial hyperplasia and cancer. For this reason, women at high risk who want to try HRT should opt for one that includes both estrogen and progesterone, rather than estrogen alone.

Blood clots: Though it is rare, HRT can increase the risk of blood clots and pulmonary embolism, especially during the first year of therapy. A family history of blood clots, obesity, and recent surgery all increase the risk and should be taken into account. Transdermal HRT (creams and patches) has a lower risk of causing blood clots than oral preparations and does not increase the risk of venous thromboembolism, so that might be a viable option.

The Benefits of HRT

HRT can help not only with current symptoms, it may also help you stay healthy and more active for decades to come. It will have the most benefit when taken within ten years of menopause. Here are some of the benefits:

Hot flashes: Hormone therapy remains the most effective FDA-approved treatment to alleviate hot flashes and night sweats. Full stop.

Sleep disorders: HRT not only helps with night sweats that can force you to change sheets in the middle of the night (not exactly restful), it can also help soothe the anxiety and mood swings that lead to tossing and turning.

Vaginal dryness: That itchy, burning, down-there discomfort? Blame it on dropping estrogen. Fifty to 60 percent of postmenopausal women experience dryness, itching, pain during intercourse, and burning when urinating. Studies have shown that systemic HRT eliminates the symptoms of vaginal atrophy in 75 percent of cases. HRT in the form of vaginal creams reduces symptoms in 80 to 90 percent of cases.

Urinary incontinence: One of the most common reasons people end up in nursing homes is urinary incontinence. In women, this is often due to a thinning of the lining of the urethra that occurs when estrogen levels drop. HRT can help to prevent this.

Osteoporosis: Loss of estrogen is the main cause of osteoporosis, which weakens bones and puts you at a greater risk for fractures, one of the main reasons women end up in nursing homes. HRT increases calcium absorption and helps protect and strengthen bones.

Heart disease: Decreasing estrogen levels contribute to the risk of cardiovascular disease, high blood pressure, changes in lipids, insulin resistance, and increased body fat that can all put a strain on your heart. According to the National Institute on Aging (NIA), "Within one year of the final menstrual period, arterial stiffness significantly increased, beyond what would be expected from aging and risk factors alone." HRT may lessen that risk and has even shown to lower total cholesterol levels. Be aware, though, that it may cause an initial bump in LDL (the "bad" cholesterol), at first, though this usually evens out.

Neurodegenerative diseases: A large meta-analysis has shown that HRT can lessen the risk of Parkinson's and Alzheimer's diseases, especially when taken during perimenopause. The benefits increase the longer you stay on it, but the duration should be balanced with the risk of other diseases. Researchers surmise that estrogen helps to protect against the deterioration of cognitive functions that occur with normal aging. The effects appear to be greatest when HRT is taken at the start of the menopausal transition, when the levels of estrogen begin to decrease. Research is ongoing about the effects when HRT is taken later on. (See Chapter 10 for information on what happens when your brain goes through estrogen withdrawal. Bottom line: It's foggy.)

Metabolic disorders: Estrogen receptors help regulate insulin, the hormone produced in the pancreas that controls the amount of glucose in your bloodstream. When estrogen levels decline, sensitivity to insulin also decreases, throwing your pancreas into overdrive and leading to too much insulin in your bloodstream. This raises the risk of metabolic syndrome, a cluster of risk factors for cardiovascular disease, inflammation, high blood pressure, and type 2 diabetes. Even women who have never had issues with prediabetes or diabetes can be affected during menopause. The increase in adipose (abdominal fat) common in menopause can further contribute to insulin resistance and increase the risk of metabolic syndrome.

HRT can help to protect against the increase in fat as well as adipose tissue inflammation and the size and number of fat cells. (See Chapters 7 and 8 on Weight and Exercise for more ways to control metabolic disorders.)

Colon cancer: In a study of over 56,000 women, HRT was shown to reduce the risk of colon cancer by up to 35 percent in postmenopausal women, even when adjusted for weight and a sedentary lifestyle and obesity (both risk factors). Researchers surmise that estrogen may inhibit tumor growth.

When to Start HRT

Every woman's experience with perimenopause and menopause, including the severity of symptoms, is different and can affect the optimal time to start HRT. That said, beginning before you turn sixty or within ten years of menopause will bring the most benefits. I often recommend women start during perimenopause when estrogen levels begin to decrease and symptoms first appear to get a head start on disease prevention. It takes approximately three months for HRT to be fully effective, but you may start feeling the benefits in as little as two to four weeks.

Andi, a forty-eight-year-old data analyst, had been in perimenopause for three years when she started HRT. "I had really low energy for a couple of years. I had joint pain and felt jittery all the time, and I wasn't sleeping, but I didn't associate it with perimenopause. I thought it was just part of getting older. Besides, I thought you had to wait until you hit menopause to start HRT. I was shocked when my doctor told me beginning now was an option. I had no idea what to expect, but I felt better within weeks. Suddenly, I was able to start functioning in a way that I thought I had lost."

Lani, fifty-nine, went into menopause when she was just forty-four. "I have endometriosis and my periods were extremely painful, so when menopause hit it was a blessing," she says. "I was lucky because I didn't suffer from hot flashes, but I began to feel as if I was outside of my body, watching myself. It felt like I was no longer a participant in my own life but experiencing it through a film of gauze. I wasn't depressed but I was no longer enjoying anything. I went back and forth about going on HRT, but when I finally started, it felt like I was finally inhabiting my own body again. I tried going off of it because I was through the worst of menopause but when the symptoms came back, I went right back on it."

Pills? Patches? Pellets? You Have Choices!

HRT is available in various forms and dosages, including pills, skin patches, vaginal rings, creams, and sprays. The choice often comes down to personal preference. Some women would rather take a daily pill, others might opt for a patch that you change weekly. For women who decide on compounded bioidentical hormones, pellets that a doctor inserts transdermally every three months are an option. In general, the goal is to use the lowest doses possible to get the desired benefits. All HRT requires a prescription, and while there are a number of options, not all are appropriate for every woman. Here are some general guidelines.

Systemic estrogen: Systemic estrogen therapy (think pills) alone—*without* progesterone—is only recommended for women not at risk for endometrial cancer who have had a hysterectomy and are suffering from hot flashes.

Transdermal estrogen: Transdermal estrogen (applied topically) in the form of a low-dose vaginal ring, gel, or cream may alleviate symptoms such as vaginal dryness without increasing the risk of blood clots or breast cancer.

Estrogen plus progesterone: For women who still have a uterus, estrogen is balanced with micronized progesterone, a newer form of the hormone that has been processed into very small particles. It is effective for treating hot flashes as well as reducing the risk of heart disease, certain cancers, and osteoporosis, and is used systemically.

Pharmaceutical, Bioidentical, and Compounded Hormones

HRT becomes even more controversial when you throw in the different ways that the hormones themselves can be formulated. There is a lot to consider—and a lot of confusion—about terminology. Let's look at the definitions of the various categories before we get into the pros and cons of each.

THE ABCS OF HRT

Pharmaceutical hormones are made by, yes, pharmaceutical companies. They use synthetic formulas of estrogen and/or progesterone in the form of tablets, patches, and gels. They are typically made from the urine of pregnant horses and are designed to have the same basic chemical makeup as the estrogen and progesterone made by your ovaries. They are regulated and approved by the FDA, are covered by insurance, and come in a limited range of doses. Examples include Premarin (just estrogen) and Prempro (estrogen plus progesterone).

Bioidentical hormones are made from plants and may include estrogen, progesterone, and testosterone. Their chemical structure is identical to that of the hormones produced by your body. The FDA has approved some (but not all) bioidentical hormone therapies for moderate to severe hot flashes. Pharmaceutical companies are increasingly bringing bioidentical hormones to the market. These are generally covered by insurance (be sure to check) and come in preformulated doses. Examples include Vivelle (just estrogen) and Prometrium (micronized progesterone).

Compounded bioidentical hormones are plant-derived bioidentical hormones that are not preformulated by a pharmaceutical company. Each doctor prescribes an individualized formula, deciding on the types of hormones and dosage based on a patient's symptoms and blood work. The prescription then goes to a compounding pharmacy where it is prepared, mixed, assembled, packaged, and labeled according to the doctor's specifications. Compounded bioidentical hormones are available in similar forms as pharmaceutical HRT including capsules, patches, creams, lozenges, and vaginal suppositories, as well as pellets that are inserted under the skin in a doctor's office. They are not FDA approved and are not covered by insurance.

Digging Into the Controversy

I use all forms of HRT in my practice: pharmaceutical, bioidentical, and compounded bioidentical hormones. I take time to lay out the pros and cons of each option for my patients to help them make a decision that they are comfortable with. I consider compounded bio-identical hormones a viable option for women and often prefer them, but because they are controversial, I want to be sure YOU understand the risks and benefits.

I'll give you the argument against them first. While many doctors think, as I do, that compounded bioidentical hormones are more natural and may be more beneficial than traditional HRT, the FDA does not guarantee their safety and they have not received the same degree of testing. The potential issues arise from the fact that compounded hormones are produced in individual pharmacies and are not subjected to the same tests for safety, efficacy, or dosing consistency as regulated HRT. This increases the risk that they might contain impurities or trace amounts of other drugs made in the same pharmacy. If you choose to use compounded bioidentical hormones, it is extremely important that you make sure your doctor works regularly with a trusted, reputable pharmacy. While the FDA doesn't approve individual compounded formulas, it does provide some oversight into the pharmacies that make them. Look for an FDA-registered compounding pharmacy that agrees to the "Good Manufacturing Processes" (GMP), to validate the potency, sterility, and stability of its medications. The pharmacy should also comply with the regulations of the state boards in its location. (Unsure? Ask, and ask again.)

Compounding is not a new feature of the drug industry. In the 1930s and 1940s, approximately 60 percent of all medications dispensed were compounded. After the rise of commercial drug manufacturers in the 1960s, compounding began to decline. Today, the practice is once again gaining popularity, largely because doctors recognize the importance of being able to customize medications. In fact, there are as many as 50,000 compounded dosage formulas dispensed every day in the U.S. The number of prescriptions of mostly unregulated compounded hormone therapy for women at menopause has reached an estimated twenty-six million to thirty-three million per year, which isn't that far off from the thirty-six million prescriptions per year for well-regulated and tested FDA-approved hormone therapy.

More research is needed, but in my opinion, bioidenticals are metabolized differently than pharmaceutical options. They more closely replicate the exact molecular structure of your body's hormones (including estrogen, testosterone, and progesterone), which leads to better absorption than the synthetic formulas.

The efficacy of compounded bioidenticals has been backed up by research. One meta-analysis found that patients reported greater satisfaction with bioidentical hormones than their synthetic counterparts. This may be due to doctors' ability to tailor the dose specifically for each patient's profile and needs. The same research indicated that bioidentical progesterone is associated with a diminished risk for breast cancer compared to synthetic progestins.

At the risk of sounding like a professor, I want to call attention to a few more studies because I know compounded bioidenticals remain a (very) touchy subject. One study found that "a daily dose significantly relieved menopausal symptoms in peri- and postmenopausal women. Cardiovascular biomarkers, inflammatory factors, immune signaling factors, and health outcomes were favorably impacted, despite very high life stress, and home and work strain in study subjects. There were no associated adverse events."

A meta-analysis of forty studies concluded that compounded vaginal hormones were found to significantly improve symptoms of vaginal atrophy. Despite the variations in absorption from different types of compounded hormones, routes, and strengths, they were consistent with FDA-approved products.

One of the biggest reasons I often prefer using compounded HRT is that it gives me the ability to personalize each patient's formula based on extensive blood panels and symptoms, rather than having to rely on the limited dosage options from pharmaceuticals. I can tweak the formula according to how a patient responds, increasing or lowering the dosage readily as needed.

While various forms of estrogen are used in different countries, the FDA only approves the use of estradiol (E2), the strongest form, for HRT in the U.S. With compounding, I have the freedom to incorporate various other forms of estrogens, including estrone (E1) and estriol (E3), which is weaker but might be better for some women, who, for instance, are experiencing strong side effects. Compounded hormones can also include progesterone, testosterone, and dehydroepiandrosterone (DHEA).

Finally, consistency is crucial to reap the benefits of HRT. I have found that some women have a tendency to forget pills and many dislike the mess of creams. For those reasons, I often use compounded bioidentical hormones in the form of pellets the size of grains of rice that are placed in the subcutaneous fat of the buttocks. This allows for steadier release of the hormones that are absorbed directly into the bloodstream, avoiding the liver and gastrointestinal system. The pellets are replaced in a doctor's office every three months. Because they are not covered by insurance, the fee is approximately $400 per dose, depending on your doctor.

Potential Side Effects

All forms of HRT have potential side effects. Some of the most common include breast tenderness, spotting, headaches, and mood swings. (Yes, these may be the same things we are trying to treat. If they persist, you might just need the dose adjusted.) Women using estrogen creams may also experience skin irritation. These issues usually resolve over time. If your side effects are severe, say if your breasts are so tender even buttoning your shirt hurts, changing the dosage may help here, too. Prescribing HRT is both a science and an art, whether you choose a pharmaceutical or bioidentical option. Often, your doctor may have to tweak the formulation, dose, and route of delivery if you are not getting the desired results,

Potential Side Effects of HRT

Approximately one out of one hundred people experience side effects from estrogen patches, gel, and spray. They include

- Headaches

- Breast pain or tenderness

- Unexpected vaginal bleeding or spotting

- Feeling sick (nausea)

- Mood changes, including low mood or depression

- Leg cramps

- Mild rash or itching

- Diarrhea

- Hair loss

Discontinuing HRT

Most women stay on HRT for four to five years and then go off it in order to lower the risk of breast cancer. There may also be changes in your overall medical status that require stopping. There are no established clinical guidelines in place about the best way to stop. While some women go cold turkey, I generally suggest tapering off over a period of months by slowly lowering the dosage they are on.

According to the *American Journal of Medicine*, "Approximately seventy-five percent of women who try to stop are able to stop without major difficulty. Although many women stop HRT without apparent problems, some who would like to quit are unable to do so, mainly because of the development of vasomotor symptoms." If hot flashes do come back, they are usually far less severe than before HRT.

The method you choose to stop does not appear to have an impact on whether or not symptoms return. If symptoms return, in all likelihood they will not be as frequent or intense, depending on how long you have been on HRT and how long it has been since your last period.

Alternatives to HRT

For women who don't want to (or can't) take hormone replacement therapy, other options can help with symptoms. Certain antidepressants, including selective serotonin reuptake inhibitors (SSRIs), may improve hot flashes and night sweats. These include citalopram (Celexa), escitalopram (Lexapro), fluoxetine (Prozac), paroxetine (Paxil), and sertraline (Zoloft). Serotonin-norepinephrine reuptake inhibitors (SNRIs) including duloxetine (Cymbalta) and venlafaxine (Effexor XR) may have the same effect. Unlike HRT, though, antidepressants do not protect against heart disease, osteoporosis, or colon cancer. A novel alternative to HRT is the use of NK3R antagonists, which are peptide neurotransmitters that work on the temperature zone in the brain to decrease hot flashes. They have been shown to decrease the frequency and severity of hot flashes.

DESIREE'S STORY

I felt like a zombie before HRT.

I was forty-seven years old when I started gaining weight and having incredible mood swings. I couldn't concentrate on anything. My whole body felt achy. My sex drive was zero. My self-confidence took a nosedive, and I didn't want to be around other people, which only made me feel worse. It was a domino effect: Was I depressed because I was too achy to exercise and was gaining weight? Was I gaining weight because I was depressed? I was embarrassed and ashamed, so I hid. I couldn't believe I'd gone up three sizes. It happened so rapidly. I didn't know how to noodle it out and I had no idea that my dropping estrogen levels could be causing this.

I tried antidepressants, but they didn't help as much as I had hoped. Finally, I had my hormone levels checked and I found out there was a reason I felt like a walking zombie. I had no estrogen! I had read negative things about HRT, but when I did more research and found out a lot of the information was old, I felt more comfortable trying it. Within weeks of starting HRT, I was standing upright again. I wish I could scream it from the mountaintops. We don't have to be out here suffering!

—Desiree Jordan, 50

Lifestyle can play a major role in alleviating symptoms. Activities including yoga, breath work, mindfulness, and meditation can help with sleep and anxiety. Studies have proven that acupuncture can help reduce hot flashes, excess sweating, mood swings, sleep disturbances, and skin and hair problems. Benefits can be felt in as little as six weeks of weekly fifteen-minute sessions. The results can last up to six months after treatments stop.

Certain foods may help as well, though the research is mostly anecdotal. Soy products contain phytoestrogens that may act like the estrogen your body produces. There is some evidence that soy products such as tofu, soy milk, and soy nuts might help with hot flashes. Herbs such as black cohosh, wild yam, dong quai, and valerian root, either in herb form or as a pill or cream, may also help with hot flashes. It's important to discuss any natural or herbal supplements, along with any medication you use, with your doctor before starting HRT, as some interaction can occur.

There is a lot to consider when it comes to HRT. No one knows your body and medical history as well as you do. No one else can decide the degree to which symptoms are impacting your quality of life. You have a right to stand by your personal preferences about whether you use HRT and what type to use. What I do urge you to do is make sure that you know all the facts. Speak to at least one doctor who is well-versed in the latest research and options available. Take all the time you need. Choice is what Generation M is all about.

CHAPTER FIVE

Will I Ever Sleep Again?

Sleep is the golden chain that ties
health and our bodies together.

—THOMAS DEKKER

Denise, forty-nine, sat in my exam room looking pale and agitated. "I swear I have an internal alarm clock that goes off at exactly 3:17 a.m. Every. Single. Night. No matter what I do, I bolt up and can never fully get back to sleep," she moaned. "How do I make it stop?"

Am I ever going to sleep again? It's a lament I hear constantly from women going through menopause. Whether you have trouble falling asleep, wake drenched in night sweats, or get zapped by anxiety on and off all night, lack of sleep can push you to the brink. It certainly doesn't help you cope with all the other changes going on. Whether it is due to hormonal changes, aging, life itself, or a tangled yarn of all three—being exhausted makes every problem seem bigger and every task more challenging.

Sleep is essential for optimal physical, cognitive, and emotional health, but as many as 50 to 60 percent of women experience some degree of insomnia during and after menopause. According to the SWAN study, sleep disorders, including the inability to fall asleep and waking up throughout the night due to hot flashes, increase with age and can affect 16 to 42 percent of premenopausal women, 39 to 47 percent of perimenopausal women, and 35 to 60 percent of post-menopausal women.

Disrupted sleep activates the sympathetic nervous system and affects the hypothalamic-pituitary-adrenocortical (HPA axis), a complex neuroendocrine system that regulates the body's response to stress by regulating metabolism, immune response, and the nervous system. Because both estrogen and progesterone help to regulate the HPA axis, when they decrease, the HPA axis gets thrown off, leading to an excess of cortisol, the stress hormone. The result? Anxiety, sleeplessness, poor concentration, and irritability. In other words, lack of restful sleep.

The short-term consequences of sleep disruption for otherwise healthy adults can include increased stress, joint and muscle pain, reduced quality of life, emotional distress, and mood disorders, along with cognitive and memory deficits. Disrupted sleep has also been found to increase the likelihood of depression.

Other long-term effects can include hypertension, changes in cholesterol levels, cardiovascular disease, weight-related issues, metabolic syndrome, type 2 diabetes mellitus, and even an increased risk of colorectal cancer.

Oh, and one more thing: if you've ever wondered why you're hungrier after a poor night's rest, it's because lack of sleep decreases levels of leptin and increases ghrelin, two hormones that regulate appetite. So, yes, insomnia can also lead to weight gain.

Before you lose more sleep worrying about losing sleep (which is definitely a thing), keep in mind that there are concrete steps you can take to improve both the quality and quantity of sleep.

What's Keeping You Up: Hormones Gone Haywire

Many things can lead to tossing and turning at night—your kids, your job, the state of the world—but hormones play a huge role. The night sweats caused by lack of estrogen certainly don't help. Lower levels of estrogen and progesterone can also lead to excess cortisol, the stress hormone. It's hard to get a good's sleep if you are consumed with worry.

The supplemental estrogen in HRT can have a beneficial effect on sleep even beyond reducing hot flashes. Studies have found that in postmenopausal women with hot flashes, night sweats, insomnia, anxiety, and mood swings, low-dose estrogen and progesterone improved sleep to a greater extent than could be explained by a reduction in vasomotor symptoms alone. In other words, what helps your mood helps your sleep.

Estrogen is not the only hormone that gets depleted during menopause. Melatonin is synthesized from serotonin, the neurohormone that promotes a feeling of calm and regulates the sleep/wake cycle. While a little melatonin is secreted during daylight hours, with the onset of darkness, melatonin synthesis and release kicks into business, peaking between two a.m. and four a.m. Unfortunately, both natural aging and menopause itself cause melatonin levels to drop in most women, leading to difficulty falling or staying asleep.

Melatonin is an over-the-counter supplement and can be worth a try, especially if you are not a candidate for HRT because of a history of breast cancer or blood clots. Melatonin has another potential benefit; it helps bones absorb calcium and may lower your risk of osteoporosis. While it is generally well tolerated, not everyone responds to it the same way. Potential side effects include dizziness, headaches, and dry mouth. While there is little research to suggest melatonin is chemically addictive, you can become psychologically dependent on it. If you decide to try it, I recommend taking no more than three milligrams per night. As with any medication or supplement, talk to your doctor first.

Sleepless Nights: Four Questions to Ask Yourself

Homing in on the root cause of why you are having trouble sleeping can lead you to the best ways to address it. Asking yourself the following four questions is a good place to start, but first talk to your doctor to rule out underlying health issues, such as restless leg syndrome, a disorder that causes an uncontrollable urge to move your legs during the night.

1. **Is this due to hot flashes?** Having to get up and change your pajamas in the middle of the night is not exactly conducive to a good night's rest. HRT is the most effective way to relieve hot flashes and night sweats. Acupuncture may also help to relieve hot flashes, increase a sense of calm, and promote better sleep quality and duration.

2. **Am I waking repeatedly in the night or having trouble breathing?** If you answered yes to this question, bring it up with your doctor. Shortness of breath or gasping in the night are symptoms of sleep apnea, a disorder in which breathing stops and starts during the night. Other symptoms include loud snoring, waking up tired, and falling asleep during the day. Sleep apnea must be diagnosed and treated by a sleep specialist. Approximately 16 percent of women over fifty develop sleep apnea, and while there is no single cause, it is tied to weight gain, which becomes more common in menopause. Sleep apnea increases the risk of heart disease but is treatable with a CPAP (continuous positive airway pressure) machine, which uses mild air pressure to keep breathing airways open while you sleep.

3. **Is my mind racing too much to fall asleep?** Extensive research has shown that practicing mindfulness, whether that entails simply focusing on your breath or meditating,

decreases sleep disturbances and improves the quality
of rest. One reason is that meditation blocks anxiety and
hyperarousal (that twitchy feeling when every nerve seems
to be firing). It can also help you process emotions, making
it less likely that you will stay awake ruminating. There are a
number of free apps that offer guided meditations specifically
geared to sleep.

4. **Do I find myself having to use the bathroom
   frequently at night?** Bladder issues, including an
   overactive bladder causing the frequent urge to pee,
   become more common in menopause and can disrupt
   sleep. HRT can reduce this in the vast majority of women.
   Another tip: Limit your liquid intake before bedtime.

Set Yourself Up for Sleep Success

Regardless of the cause of insomnia, there are lifestyle hacks that
will up your chances of a good night's sleep. If you have a partner,
your tossing and turning is probably affecting them, too. Have an
open conversation about the changes you are going through and the
lifestyle changes you plan to make.

The first change, which you probably know but bears repeating, is to limit caffeine. While the stimulant effects can be felt within
thirty minutes, caffeine stays in your body for hours. I recommend
stopping all caffeine, including coffee, black tea, and most sodas, by
twelve p.m. It is also a good idea to stop eating three hours before

bedtime. This gives your body time to digest food, reducing the risk of acid reflux or bloating that might wake you up.

Screen time is another thing you should put the brakes on at least one hour before bedtime. The blue light from screens can fool your body into thinking it's daytime, and thus suppresses the production of the sleep-inducing hormone melatonin. Plus, doom-scrolling has never helped anyone fall asleep. Ever. If you wake in the middle of the night, resist the urge to pick up your phone to distract yourself. In fact, leave your phone in another room. (I admit I have a hard time with this one, but I'm working on it.) Try using a good old digital clock for an alarm instead of your phone.

Getting in the habit of journaling in the evening can help you sort out any troubling emotions that have the tendency to come back to haunt you the minute the lights go off. Writing a to-do list for the next day can also keep you from feeling overwhelmed or worrying that you will forget something important.

If you are prone to night sweats, keep an extra pair of pajamas handy so you don't have to turn on the lights and rummage around. Finally, hot flashes or not, keeping the thermostat in your bedroom around sixty-five degrees can help regulate your body temperature and promote deeper sleep.

Strike a Pose for Better Sleep

Not only is yoga one of the best forms of exercise for strength and flexibility, but it can also increase sleep quality and duration, especially

BUILDING BLOCK

Tame Your "Worry Brain"

Daytime worries have a nasty tendency to mushroom the minute the lights go out. My friend Dr. Christiane Wolf, who shared her tips on how to begin a meditation practice with us earlier, has advice on how to deal with what she calls "Worry Brain" at night. When you find your thoughts going in circles, she suggests taking these four steps to tame the anxiety and bring on the calm that leads to better sleep.

1. Become aware: Turn toward your concern instead of away.

We often unconsciously push our experience aside or even pretend it's not happening. Instead, turn toward the situation that's troubling you in a focused way. Don't dwell on it, but acknowledge it. That simple act will bring a greater sense of perspective and control.

2. Name it, tame it, and distance yourself from it.

The "name it to tame it" strategy is popular in psychotherapy. Research has shown that when we name what we are going through, we gain a healthy sense of distance between ourselves and the experience. For example, instead of thinking *I am worried,* name the experience as an object. *There is worry* or *There is worry in my mind.* That allows you to observe it without judgment.

3. Switch channels.

Worry is often experienced as racing thoughts, but it is also felt in the body—for example, as tightness in the chest. When you are in a nonstop cycle of worried thoughts, it's hard to think yourself out of it. What helps is to "switch the channel" to *sensing* rather than *thinking*. Concentrate on the breath going through your nostrils. How does it feel? Where is it going? How does the exhalation feel? Do this for one minute and repeat as necessary when your attention goes back to thinking rather than feeling.

4. Be kind to yourself.

Speak to yourself as you would a friend. Try telling yourself, "Having worry mind is hard." Or, "Going through menopause is hard." It can help to put your hand on your heart as you do this to feel a tactile sense of kindness.

in perimenopause and menopause when stress takes a toll. "Focusing on breathing and conscious relaxation can lower your heart rate and blood pressure," says my friend Gabrielle Espinosa, a yoga instructor and menopause and sexual wellness coach. "It switches our parasympathetic nervous system into 'rest and restore,' which brings a sense of calm and allows us to change the way we perceive and respond to stress."

Save fast-paced classes that raise your heart rate for daytime. In the evening, opt for slower hatha yoga or yoga nidra, which focuses on breathing and restorative poses that include lying or sitting down. (See Chapter 8, "The Exercise Rx," for more on specific types of yoga.)

Get Moving

Thirty minutes of moderate exercise (think brisk walking) during the day can help reduce the time it takes you to fall asleep. If you did have a restless night, getting your body moving—even if it's just a short stroll outside—can give you a burst of much-needed energy and help clear your head. As a bonus, exercise can help to control weight gain, one of the causes of sleep apnea.

Try Cognitive Behavioral Therapy (CBT)

We've already seen how CBT is a science-backed therapy approach that can help you change negative emotions associated with menopause.

It can also help you reduce sleep-related anxiety and is an effective way to control insomnia. An example of sleep-related anxiety? Lying awake worrying about how tired you will be the next day. CBT trains you to replace negative thoughts about sleep with more positive, realistic messaging along the lines of *I will be able to function tomorrow even if I'm a little tired.*

Along with rewiring your thought patterns around insomnia, CBT teaches behaviors that promote better sleep. One important tip: get out of bed after twenty minutes if you are unable to fall asleep, and don't return until you are sleepy. This will train your body and mind to associate bed with rest, not restlessness. Other CBT techniques include creating a regular sleep schedule. That means even if you have trouble falling asleep, you shouldn't change your wake-up time or nap the next day. Keeping a sleep diary where you track your progress will help you recognize and change unhelpful behaviors. CBT is not just about what you "shouldn't" do. It teaches relaxation techniques, including deep breathing and guided imagery.

CBT is usually done with a therapist and takes about three to four weeks to be effective to improve sleep. While meeting in-person with an expert in CBT is great, it is not necessary. In a study published in *JAMA Internal Medicine* that specifically targeted women with menopausal sleep problems, six CBT therapy sessions via telephone over an eight-week period improved sleep. Internet-based courses in CBT have also been shown to be effective.

CBT curious? The U.S. Department of Veterans Affairs has created a free app, "The Insomnia Coach," that can walk you through the basics and help you create your own sleep journal.

GWENDOLYNE'S STORY

Do I start taking gummies? Drink tea?

I'm in the middle of perimenopause and started getting night sweats about two years ago. Suddenly, I realized why people spend so much money on sheets! On top of the hormonal changes, I have three kids, and my mind was racing at night. I had to figure out a better way to take care of myself, but I had no idea what that would look like. Do I start taking gummies? Drink tea?

What helped me was meditation and learning to give space to my brain. I realized that if I sat still, I was just as powerful as if I was moving. With the stress I was going through and changes in my body, meditation allowed me to be okay with who I am, to understand that I am a human having a human experience. It allows me to step aside in a lot of situations and say, *Okay, how I handle this is a choice.* I don't think I ever gave myself the space to do that. I realized that if you're not taking care of your own greatness, then you're not going to be able to give other people what they need. Giving myself the space to do that is one of the most important things I do.

It helped me cope better during the day and eased my anxiety so I could fall asleep at night. Oh, and bamboo sheets make a big difference, too!

—Gwendolyne Osbourne, 45

Do a Nighttime Body Scan

A great way to calm your mind, reduce anxiety, and promote sleep is to do a body scan meditation while lying in bed that helps you focus on physical sensations rather than spinning thoughts. In bed with the lights off, concentrate on how your feet feel on the mattress. How do your toes feel? What do the sheets beneath your ankles feel like? Move on to your legs, your knees, and all the way up to your head, taking deep breaths at each place. How does each body part feel? What sensations are you experiencing? Be curious and non-judgmental, and go slow. If you find your mind wandering, that's natural. Just start again. A body scan can take ten minutes or longer.

Think Before You Take Sleep Medication

I always recommend trying lifestyle changes first before considering sleep medications. That said, they are among the most prescribed medications in America. There are a growing range of prescription options, from zolpidem (Ambien) to ramelteon (Rozerem) to suvorexant (Belsomra), designed to help you fall and stay asleep. Be aware that all have potential side effects ranging from dizziness to headaches and confusion. They are not meant for long-term use, and you may experience withdrawal symptoms when you stop. As with any drugs, talk to your doctor about different types of sleep medication available, side effects, and potential interactions with other drugs.

CHAPTER SIX

Reclaiming Your Libido

Real intimacy is only possible to the degree that we can be honest about what we are doing and feeling.

—JOYCE BROTHERS

Joannie sat across from me, fidgeting nervously. She was a new patient and seemed comfortable talking openly about medical history—until I brought up her sex life. Her eyes narrowed and she looked at me warily. "Why are you asking?" she demanded. I explained that it is a question I ask every patient. "This is a judgment-free zone," I assured her. "I don't care how many partners you have or don't have. I don't care what your preferences are, but intimacy is an important part of life. If there are problems, it's something we should discuss."

It wasn't until Joannie's follow-up visit two weeks later that she trusted me enough to admit that she was avoiding sex with her husband because it had become too painful. "I feel like my insides are ripping apart," she said as she began to cry, "but I'm scared my husband will leave me for a younger woman." I listened while she poured out her fears. When she was calmer, I promised her that we would find ways to deal with the pain, not because she was worried that her husband might leave her, but because she has a *right* to a pleasurable sex life. We all do, and as part of Generation M, we owe it to ourselves to own that.

Many women experience changes to their sex lives during perimenopause and menopause, from loss of libido to painful intercourse. Despite how common the phenomenon is, it can be hard to talk openly about it. Our society still stigmatizes women's right to express desire, especially at this stage of life. For so long, we have been given the message overtly and subliminally that women over a certain age are not viable sexual beings. That once we are no longer fertile, we are no longer useful. Yes, there are physical and psychological changes that occur as we age. There are also adjustments we can make to deal with them. I'm not saying you have to have a rollicking sex life (though go right ahead if that works for you) or expect to have the same roaring libido you had at eighteen. Sex, like everything in life, changes as we get older. That doesn't mean it has to vanish. Sexuality, desire, and desirability exist on a continuum well past menopause. There is no reason you can't have a fully satisfying intimate life for decades to come.

Not every doctor will ask you about your sex life, but I urge you to bring it up if you are experiencing any changes or pain. There are proactive steps you can take, including hormone replacement therapy and lubricants that lessen discomfort during intercourse. There are techniques, too, that can help you have an open conversation with your partner and feel more in touch with your own body.

"I encourage women at every age to approach sex with a sense of joy," says my friend Dr. Nan Wise, PhD, a neuroscientist, bestselling author, sex therapist, and licensed psychotherapist. "During and after the menopausal transition, our sex lives can actually improve. With a little work, we can have a better relationship with ourselves, let go of hang-ups that hold us back, and enjoy sex in completely new ways. Yes, we are older and our bodies have changed, but experience gives us the wisdom to be more honest with ourselves. That can be a real turn-on and lead to deep, sustainable relationships. It's about creating a new leg of the journey. I know from my professional and personal experience, it's never too late to have a blooming sex life."

Let's Get Physical: Hormones and Libido, Pain and Pleasure

Geri, now fifty-one, enjoyed a good sex life up until her mid-forties, even with two teenagers at home. "When perimenopause hit, everything suddenly dried up," she says. "Sex was painful. I had no libido at all and felt no pleasure when we did have sex. Intimacy is important to me, and I felt like I was failing. My husband, Jim, and I went to a couples therapist, who helped him understand that my loss of libido wasn't because I didn't love him but that my hormones were wreaking havoc. I had seen my regular OB/GYN but she never asked

Unraveling the Road Blocks to Intimacy

Issues pertaining to sex and intimacy can feel overwhelming. A good way to untangle what you are going through is to ask yourself probing questions about your physical, psychological, and emotional sexual well-being. The answers can help guide you to the right treatments. Use the following questions as prompts for journaling.

1. Has your level of desire changed?

2. Has the frequency of your intimacy changed?

3. When you are in the midst of intimate moments, including intercourse, do you enjoy it?

4. Do you have pain during intercourse?

5. Have your thoughts on sexual intimacy changed?

6. Has the nature of your orgasm changed?

about my sex life, and I didn't bring it up. Finally, I switched to a new doctor who was very direct. She asked me what was going on down there and explained vaginal atrophy to me, which was making sex painful. She helped me understand that my lack of libido was normal, not a personal failing. Intimacy is not something I wanted to sacrifice, and she made it a priority to figure out solutions, including changing the dose of HRT I was on."

There are probably no two less sexy words in the English language than "vaginal atrophy." Unfortunately, though, menopause does cause structural changes to the vagina that can make sex painful. The decrease in estrogen can lead to genitourinary syndrome of menopause (GSM), a myriad of diagnoses that impact the labia, clitoris, vagina, and lower urinary tract. (A side note: the term "vaginal atrophy" has proved so distasteful that it has largely been simply replaced by "GSM.") Among the results are thinning and dryness in the vaginal lining. That's what causes women like Geri to experience discomfort during sex, including irritation, burning, and even bleeding after intercourse. As a first step, I recommend trying lubricants, especially if you are on the fence about estrogen supplementation. Water or silicone-based lubricants can help decrease the friction that causes discomfort.

Some of my patients find silicone irritating, and it may take some experimentation to find what works best for you. "I have always been playful and expressive sexually," Stacy, fifty-one, says. "It was a happy area of my life. I had just started dating a new man when menopause hit, and sex was excruciating. My libido and ability to orgasm didn't change, but it felt as if I was tearing every time we tried. Luckily, my guy handled it well. We tried various lubricants, but I didn't want to smell like a Jolly Rancher. We found coconut oil was the best."

Stacy was lucky, but many women experience a change to how they orgasm. The lining of the vagina and vulva are rich in estrogen receptors. Dropping estrogen levels can cause a decrease in blood flow and the secretions that impact pleasure, arousal, and the intensity of orgasm. Hormone replacement therapy, whether pharmaceutical or bioidentical, can be beneficial at reducing dryness and pain and increasing blood flow and pleasure for many women.

Some women have found taking testosterone supplements can improve arousal and their ability to orgasm. A large study published in the *British Journal of General Practice* found that, "In post-menopausal women, testosterone supplementation improved several domains of sexual response, including sexual desire, pleasure, arousal, orgasm, and self-image. It has also been shown to have additional benefits, including the improvement of urogenital, psychological, and somatic symptoms, an increase in bone density, and enhancement of cognitive performance when combined with estrogen as part of HRT. Many women notice that taking testosterone improves their mood, concentration, motivation, and energy levels."

Before you consider testosterone, it is important to talk to a doctor well-versed in its usage. When dosages are too high, side effects can include excess body hair and acne. It can take several weeks to months to feel the full effect. It is often safer to use a low dose and have levels tested regularly. One word of warning: There is not enough research to know whether testosterone supplementation is safe for women with, or at high risk for, breast cancer. (See Chapter 4: "The ABCs of HRT.")

There are ways to improve physical sensation without hormones. Doing Kegel exercises can help strengthen the pelvic floor, which can improve sexual sensations and may help with urinary incontinence. Finally, there is the option of vaginal rejuvenation with CO_2 lasers to reduce dryness, improve elasticity, and improve urinary incontinence.

BUILDING BLOCK
The Kegel Effect

Kegel exercises, in which you tighten the pelvic floor, have a reputation of being the post-pregnancy must-do, but they are also important before, during, and after menopause to strengthen the pelvic floor muscles and prevent urinary incontinence. Practice tightening your pelvic floor muscles to the count of ten. How do you know if you are finding the right muscles? Try stopping the flow of urine while you are peeing. It's the same muscles. I recommend doing them several times a day (no one needs to know!). You should see results in two to four weeks.

In a clinical setting, a probe is inserted into the vagina, allowing a laser to focus heat on the surrounding tissue, spurring collagen and elastin production. The procedure usually requires two to three twenty-minute treatments spaced four to six weeks apart. While it is often performed by a dermatologist, you should always see your gynecologist first about any safety concerns. It is not covered by insurance and can cost between two thousand and four thousand dollars.

Getting in the Mood

The emotional swings of perimenopause and menopause can also take a toll on your libido. Decreasing hormone levels can affect your energy, mood, and sleep patterns, all of which have an impact on desire. If you're exhausted from insomnia or worried about having hot flashes in the middle of the night, it's hard to feel sexy.

Worrying about what you look like doesn't help either. It can take time to come to peace with the changes your body is going through, whether that means some extra pounds around your middle or new lines around your eyes. Feeling insecure can make you less likely to initiate sex or be able to lose yourself in the moment.

These are not simple things to get over, as much as I wish they were. I do know that you are probably far harder on yourself than your partner is. I also know that comparing yourself to unrealistic body standards is a buzzkill.

Tuning in to physical sensations can help you get away from viewing your body negatively and see it as a source of pleasure. It's not about a simplistic mantra of "love your body." Instead, try a somatic (holistic) practice that helps you get out of your head and into your body. Start by paying attention to how you experience sensations throughout the day. *How does movement feel? What tastes good? What touch do I like?* You are training yourself to concentrate on how your body *feels* rather than dwelling on negative thoughts. With practice, that can carry over into more intimate moments.

Getting Out of a Sexual Rut

Having a "date night" is a cliché by now, but that's because it works. It is all too easy when you are dealing with menopausal symptoms,

BUILDING BLOCK
Exercise for Better Sex

A sedentary lifestyle is not good for any aspect of physical or psychological health, including your sexual life. Getting moving (outside the bedroom) can increase activity in the sympathetic nervous system, which is involved in arousal and orgasm. Exercise also stimulates oxytocin and cortisol, and can spur estrogen, all of which benefit sexual function. Strength training may also boost testosterone, which increases sex drive. Throw in some ab work, too. A strong core improves balance and stamina, and allows you to be a bit more, shall we say, experimental when it comes to positions.

Not up for picking up the weights? Because low levels of vitamin D have been associated with decreased sexual desire and pleasure, going for a fifteen-minute walk in the sun is a great way to boost your fitness level and your libido. As with all exercise, talk to your doctor first—and then get moving.

balancing a job and home life, to put sex on the back burner. You don't have to aim for a specific frequency, but if sex is a priority for you, make sure you allow time for it, even if it means letting a few other to-do's slide.

Trying new positions can keep things interesting. While you might not be able to perform the athletic moves you once did (your "flinging each other across the bed" days may be over), that doesn't mean you can't find new routes to satisfaction that take any changes in flexibility or physical limitations into account. I often recommend couples go to a sex therapist for help navigating the physical and emotional issues that can hold us back from approaching sex with a sense of joy and play. You are about to hear from one of my favorites, Dr. Nan Wise, PhD, a neuroscientist and sex therapist.

Dealing with a Desire Discrepancy

It is natural for desire to wax and wane if you are in a long-term relationship, especially as menopausal symptoms intensify. Being open with your partner can prevent a desire discrepancy from causing a deeper rift. Mary, a forty-nine-year-old office manager in Kentucky, sensed that her husband had begun to worry about her lack of libido. "We've only been married for six years, so you'd think my desire would be stronger, but to be honest, sex just never crosses my mind," she says. "My husband felt rejected, and it was causing issues in our marriage. He is in the medical field and when we both realized that my loss of desire was due to hormones, not anything either of us was doing wrong, it gave us a less emotionally loaded way to think about it."

If you are experiencing a desire discrepancy, Dr. Wise suggests opening the topic with your partner in a neutral setting. "Show that you understand their point of view," she suggests. "You might say something along the lines of *I know this is a bummer for you. Let's think of things we can do together that might add more fun.* It doesn't necessarily have to be intercourse. The goal is to create a system of give and take, seeking and engaging, getting curious and exploring.

Having that approach to your partnership will keep communication open. Libidos are ever-fluctuating, and a discrepancy now doesn't mean it will stay that way forever, but you want to keep the connection going."

Talking to Your Partner: Get Comfortable with Discomfort

"The number one sex issue, even more than loss of desire, is people not talking to each other," Dr. Wise says. "If you recognize that it's not only okay to feel uncomfortable with being open about your sexuality, but that learning to tolerate those feelings is an important life skill, you can lean into the discomfort. Taking the risk and entering into these conversations can transform embarrassment and shame into enthusiasm and excitement, and bring a new level of connection with your partner."

Ren, a banker in Texas, struggled having that conversation. "It took me a while to figure out how to talk to my husband about what was going on," she says. "We'd always had an equal interest in sex, but that changed. I never initiated sex anymore. It was too uncomfortable for me. One night, my husband took me out for a date night, and I looked across the table from him and said, 'I want you to understand what's going on for me. I have no drive, no impulse, no desire to have sex with you, or with anybody for that matter.' I didn't want him to feel unloved or undesired. I was trying to explain to him that I felt like I could happily become a nun. I didn't feel desirable. Once I made it clear what I was going through, he looked at me and said, 'We will deal with this together.' That really helped. I told him I wanted him to keep trying to initiate while still understanding my feelings. He is such a gracious and kind person. It took time and hormones and lubricants, but we got there."

You can increase your comfort level with The Talk by learning specific communication tools. "When you are approaching any fraught relationship topic, I recommend a slow start-up, rather than jumping right in," Dr. Wise says. "You can start by saying to your partner something like, *Honey, there's something I'm really uncomfortable about bringing up with you. Do you have the space and energy to talk about it now, or should we set it up for later today or tomorrow?* Letting your partner know your intention can lessen the chance of them feeling ambushed. Setting up a private time to talk will also give both of you time to gather your thoughts and set a clear intention for what you want to say."

Dr. Wise suggests framing the conversation in a positive light to avoid putting your partner on the defensive. "One way to do that is to say, *I want to talk about this because I want us to be able to have more fun together.* Putting the focus on fun rather than directly on sex can avoid framing the conversation in a negative light. Try not to fixate on what you think your sex life is "supposed" to look like, but rather, make it about getting excited about going to the playground with your partner again."

Be specific about any physical and emotional changes you are going through, whether it's hot flashes, sleep disturbance, or vaginal dryness. That can help you find ways to integrate changes, whether it's a new position or a new time, that might help. If you are having difficulty, or feel like your needs are not being met, talk to a sex and intimacy coach. Going together can help your partner understand the transition you are going through and learn new ways to be supportive.

One word of caution: Alcohol may give you the "liquid courage" to have difficult conversations, but it can lessen your sensitivity to touch and impair your ability to orgasm. A meta-analysis of over 50,000 women found that alcohol reduces sensitivity to touch, resulting in decreased libido, arousal, and intensity. It can also cause delays in achieving orgasm and reduce blood flow to the genital area, leading to vaginal dryness.

Dating While Hot

Dating is hard enough without worrying that you are going to have a hot flash in the middle of your first dinner. It takes motivation to put yourself out there and meet someone new. Blake, fifty-three, started dating soon after getting a divorce. "I was lucky to meet a man who was fifty-six and married before, so he was probably a bit more understanding," she says. "I had to tell him what I was going through. There's no hiding night sweats if I have to get up and change the sheets because they're soaked. Once I opened up, it became far less awkward. We can laugh about it. Plus, it's actually a relief not to have to worry about getting pregnant."

Dr. Wise suggests checking in with yourself before embarking on a dating quest to be sure it is what you really want and not something you just *think* you should be doing. Once you are clear on your answer, she says, "Go out there and sweat and be authentic." While

LANI'S STORY

I have a young hot husband, but no libido for the first time ever.

I did not have any overt signs of perimenopause that I was aware of. I have endometriosis, which makes every period very painful. I was forty-four years old when they stopped completely, and it was a blessing for me. The downside was that I had just married a man who was eight years younger than me, and suddenly I was in menopause. I called up a friend who warned me not to use the word "menopause" with my new husband. She warned it would be a complete turnoff. My sexuality had always been an important part of my life, but I didn't say a word. The problem was that despite having a young hot husband, I had no libido for the first time ever. When we had sex it was fine, but it wasn't like I woke up the next morning and wanted to do it again. I finally went on HRT and began to feel spicy and more present. I accept that I will never have the same sex drive I did earlier in my life, but it is important to me and to my marriage to keep that connection. The funny thing is, when I got up the nerve to tell my husband, it was no big deal at all. I think he knew but didn't want to say anything until I brought it up.

—Lani, 54

it may be uncomfortable (as dating often is), being open about where you are coming from, including your menopause journey, can be a litmus test to find out if the other person is someone who will really be there for you.

Prime the Pump

"If you're not regularly priming the pump, it's very easy to lose access to libido," Dr. Wise says. Rather than going into "sexual retirement," she recommends intentionally jump-starting your sex drive. "Sometimes, the best thing to do whether you feel like it or not is using a vibrator to have an orgasm. You don't have to feel bad about coercing yourself to have sex if it's going to be helpful. You are priming the pump and getting back into your sensations. An added bonus is that there will be a natural release of testosterone, which is responsible for the sex drive in both men and women."

Before you panic that sex will never be sexy again, not every woman experiences a loss of libido. Jenny, fifty-three, found herself in the thick of menopause two years after her husband died. "He was my high school sweetheart, but he had been sick for so long that in many ways I had already gone through a lot of the grieving process," she says. "He was my whole world, and dating was very new to me. I am bisexual, so that broadens the field. It is challenging that so many people my age are already coupled up, but I keep trying, because if anything, my libido has gone up, which I wasn't expecting. I laugh because I buy more batteries for my vibrator now than I did when I was younger."

CHAPTER SEVEN

Weight, What?

Be happy in your own skin. If you are
unhealthy, start by making small changes
to become healthier. You are unique,
beautiful, and worthy.

—OCTAVIA SPENCER

Deirdre, fifty, a special ed teacher in Ohio, was so embarrassed about gaining eighteen pounds that she started making excuses to avoid seeing people socially, even her oldest friends. "It was like I woke up one day with this giant fluffy pillow wrapped around my waist. I couldn't fit into any of my clothes. I was ashamed that I had let myself go. The more depressed I got, the less active I became, and the more weight I put on. It felt like my body was betraying me," she says.

Show me a woman who doesn't have a tangled emotional relationship with weight, and I will show you a unicorn. I wish that wasn't the case, but we're here to be real. And we're here to change that.

We are trained almost from birth to tie our self-worth to a number on the scale or a certain jeans size. We are taught that thin bodies are the ideal at every age. We see weight loss glorified almost every time we turn on the television or open our social media accounts. The discussion of weight in our society is rarely tied to *health*; instead, it is treated instead as a measure of desirability. We assume gaining weight shows a lack of discipline. It can be especially frustrating if you are eating and exercising the same way you have in the past but the pounds pile up regardless.

Internalizing societal pressures about body size can not only lead to depression, but also result in unhealthy dieting and/or binge eating that will harm your emotional and physical well-being. Above all, it holds women back from concentrating on what matters most when it comes to their weight and improving their health, longevity, and confidence. It's time Generation M stops this cycle of self-blame.

The unavoidable fact is that your metabolism changes during perimenopause and menopause.

Approximately 60 to 70 percent of women experience weight gain in midlife. Muscle mass naturally declines with age for most people, in part because we tend to become more sedentary. For women, hormonal changes can decrease lean muscle mass and tip the fat-to-muscle ratio in the wrong direction. Even if your weight doesn't change, the way it is distributed is likely to. These are biological facts, but understanding them intellectually and accepting them emotionally can be two very different things.

If I have one wish for Generation M (okay, I have more than one but let's start here), it is that we change the lens to view weight—and weight maintenance—as one element in the broader picture of life-long health. While I'm all in favor of a little vanity if that motivates you to make changes, the larger goal is to have more energy and strength, and to reduce the risk of chronic disease.

The Meno Metabolism Riddle

Because there are estrogen receptors in your muscles, when hormone levels dip, the muscles themselves grow smaller and weaker. The metabolic rate of muscles (how quickly they burn calories) is three times higher than that of fat. In other words, the more muscle you have, the higher your metabolism will be. You will burn calories more efficiently even at rest. I'm not talking about bulking up like a superhero, but the math is undeniable. Unless you take proactive steps to protect, and increase, your muscle mass, fat will begin to accumulate, particularly around your middle. (See Chapter 8, "The Exercise Rx," for how to get started.) There's another reason that loss of muscle causes weight gain. Muscles use glucose as their main source of energy. When muscle declines, the unused sugar floods the bloodstream, leading to insulin resistance, and, often, the cravings for more sugar and high-fat carbohydrates that pack on pounds. As we will see, strength training, eating more protein, getting enough sleep, cutting back on sugar, and HRT can help to combat the menopausal metabolism riddle.

Decreasing levels of estrogen shift how and where we store fat. Postmenopausal women in general have twice as much visceral fat than premenopausal women, which accumulates around the middle and can be detrimental to your health. Unlike subcutaneous fat, which is found just beneath the skin (the kind you can pinch), visceral fat wraps around organs in the abdominal cavity, including your liver, pancreas, and intestines.

Too much visceral fat can lead to metabolic syndrome, a group of conditions including high blood pressure, high cholesterol or triglyceride levels, heart disease, and stroke. Along with the specific health risks of visceral fat, being overweight in general can make menopausal symptoms, including cardiovascular risk, bladder health, and even hot flashes, worse. That said, there are some changes you may just have to accept.

Nina, a marketing executive in New Jersey, found she had to change how she dressed even though she hadn't gained weight. "I cut way back on sugar, I don't eat unhealthily, but everything began to shift around by the time I turned forty-five," she says. "There's a softness in my belly I never had before. I stopped tucking shirts into my jeans and wearing anything tight, but I have to admit, it's frustrating."

There Are No Quick Fixes

I am not a proponent of fad diets, fasts, or eating plans that are overly restrictive. Not only do they have the potential to negatively impact your metabolism in the long run, but any diet that requires ongoing deprivation is not sustainable. Deducting too many calories can also lead to decreased libido and a weakened immune system, both things we are trying to build up, not tear down.

Many of my patients ask about weight loss drugs. While there are promising medications coming on the market that have the potential to help with weight loss and diseases associated with obesity, there is no blanket yes or no answer. So much depends on your medical history and lifestyle. I suggest you consult with your physician if you are interested in them and discuss whether they are an appropriate option.

Rather than quick fixes, I strongly believe that implementing small changes in how you exercise, eat, and drink is the most effective way to maintain your weight, improve your health, and reduce the risk of chronic diseases.

Don't Skip Meals

"The reality is that our metabolic rate slows as we age. That is something that nobody can escape," Tamar Samuels says. "There are things we can do to optimize our metabolic rate, including eating more protein and doing strength training, but skipping meals is not one of them. Going too long without eating forces your body to store energy, which slows your metabolism even further. It also increases cortisol, the stress hormone, which signals to your metabolism that you are in starvation mode and raises blood glucose levels, increasing hunger as well as risk of type 2 diabetes." Not only that, but high cortisol levels lead to an accumulation of unhealthy abdominal fat, the very thing you are trying to avoid. "To keep your metabolism humming, it is more effective to eat small meals every four hours or so," Samuels suggests. "For most women, that translates into three main meals and a healthy snack. Including protein in every meal will further help to regulate your appetite and slow the absorption of carbohydrates."

Pump up the Protein

Along with strength training, which we will talk about in the upcoming chapter on exercise, increasing your intake of protein, which is a key building block of muscle, is one of the most effective ways to offset the metabolic changes that occur during menopause.

Because protein takes longer to digest than carbohydrates, it stays in your stomach longer, keeping you full. It also has a higher thermic effect (the rate of energy needed to digest, absorb, and distribute the nutrients of food) than carbohydrates or fat. That means your body has to use more calories to digest protein than other foods, further boosting your metabolism. Other high thermic foods include beans, nuts, seeds, and whole grains.

Increasing your protein intake has other benefits specific to menopause. Protein is an important source of amino acids, which help maintain bone density and offset osteoporosis. One amino acid in particular, leucine, passes the blood/brain barrier faster than others, which may help regulate moods and slow cognitive decline.

There are various ways to get the optimal amount of protein, whether you are an omnivore, vegetarian, or vegan. There are differences, though. Meat is considered a "complete protein" because it contains the nine essential amino acids that help break down food, boost your immune system, and grow and repair body tissues and muscles. (There are twenty amino acids in total, but these are considered the most important.) That doesn't mean you should eat red meat with every meal, which is not necessarily good for the environment or your overall health. Personally, I eat meat in moderation (around three times a week), but I would never tell someone who is a vegetarian or vegan to change.

It is possible to get all of the protein you need from plants, dairy, beans, whole grains, seeds, and nuts, but they don't all contain the same number or type of amino acids. A few non-meat foods that are considered "complete proteins" include pea protein (good to mix into smoothies) and soy. To make sure you are getting the full range of essential amino acids, think about getting them from combining foods rather than a single source, for instance brown rice and beans or lentils. (Grains have amino acids, just different ones than meat.)

The most recent dietary guidelines for Americans recommend that healthy adults consume 10 to 35 percent of their calories a day from protein. For weight loss, getting 25 to 30 percent of calories from protein may be more effective.

Don't aim to get all your protein in one meal. Eating foods with protein throughout the day will help you keep your energy up. You can start by swapping bread or pastries at breakfast for eggs or Greek yogurt with berries. For lunch and dinner, add a protein serving that is about the size of your palm, whether that is fish, chicken, lean meat, or tofu.

Even if you don't go full-out vegetarian, eating a more plant-based diet can have strong health benefits during menopause. Studies show that eating less red meat can lower the risk of breast cancer in postmenopausal women as well as help to offset the heightened risk of heart disease, diabetes, and colon cancer. The benefits are even greater if you eliminate highly processed meats (hot dogs, for instance) that contain saturated fatty acids.

Making sure you get a good amount of your protein from nuts, legumes, and whole grains has other benefits, too. They contain high amounts of antioxidant and anti-inflammatory compounds that may help reduce menopausal symptoms. Soy can be particularly helpful in reducing the frequency and severity of hot flashes. Leafy greens and tofu are rich in calcium and can help prevent osteoporosis.

Cut Back on Sugar (Yes, There Are Ways to Make It Easier)

Because insulin resistance is more common in perimenopause and menopause, managing sugar consumption is particularly important at this time of life to prevent type 2 diabetes. Eating (or drinking) sugar also causes spikes, and crashes, in energy, which can worsen menopausal fatigue and irritability. If you need one more reason to cut back, sugar is pro-inflammatory and increases the risk of chronic disease over the time.

"Sugar doesn't have any real nutritional value," Tamar Samuels says. "It's what we call 'energy dense,' which means that it's high in calories and low in nutrients, so you're not getting much bang for your buck. Nutrient dense foods, on the other hand, contain a lot of vitamins, minerals, phytonutrients for not a lot of calories."

The goal isn't to avoid sugar completely, but to cut back. This can be especially difficult if you have been eating a diet high in sugar,

BUILDING BLOCK

Ten High-Protein Foods to Add to Your Diet

As you get older, your body needs more protein to maintain lean muscle mass. Because protein helps you stay full longer, it can also be helpful in weight maintenance. Here are some high-protein foods to add into your diet.

1. 3-ounce chicken breast: 27 grams of protein

2. 1 cup of cottage cheese: 23 grams of protein

3. 1 can of tuna fish: 22 grams of protein

4. 3 ounces fish: 17 grams of protein (while all fish is good, of course, salmon, tilapia, and mackerel are standouts)

5. 5 ounces Greek yogurt: 12 to 18 grams of protein

6. 3 ounces tofu: 9 grams of protein

7. ½ cup lentils: 9 grams of protein

8. 2 tablespoons peanut butter: 7 grams of protein

9. 1 egg: 6 to 8 grams of protein

10. ¼ cup walnuts or almonds: 4 to 6 grams of protein

which makes cravings more intense and alters your taste buds, raising the threshold for what you perceive as sweet. Along with slowing down your metabolism, skipping meals increases sugar cravings. Instead, opt for balanced meals that include protein and healthy fats that leave you feeling satisfied. When a craving hits, dark chocolate is a terrific treat to reach for. It is high in antioxidants and flavonoids that may lower blood pressure and cholesterol, and reduce the risk of heart disease. Recent studies show that it may even help prevent cognitive decline. Because dark chocolate is lower in sugar than other desserts or candy, it is less likely you'll overdo it.

Reducing added sugar to below six teaspoons a day and limiting sugary drinks to less than one full serving a week can reduce the negative effects on your health. Here are some ways to make that easier.

- **Read labels.** You don't need to be a detective to know that cookies have sugar, but it also lurks in many foods you may not expect to find it in. Some surprising culprits: instant oatmeal, many prepared tomato sauces, fruit yogurts (though you can find ones with less sugar), many granola and protein bars, packaged bread, and prepared salad dressings. Instead, try alternatives such as natural peanut butter and applesauce with no added sugars.

- **Sensitize your palate.** There are two approaches to taming sugar cravings: going cold turkey for a set amount of time (say, two weeks) or a gradual reduction. Eliminating sugar for a couple of weeks can sensitize your palate. As you slowly reintroduce (small) amounts of sugar back into your diet, you may find your taste buds have become more sensitized. Foods you loved suddenly taste too sweet, leading you to want much less sugar overall. Other people find they can get a similar result by gradually cutting back. If you add sugar to coffee or use it when baking, start by halving the amount you typically use.

- **Try sweet alternatives.** Whether you go cold turkey or gradually cut back, there are ways to satisfy a sweet craving without added sugar. Try adding fresh fruit, including berries and bananas, cinnamon, and vanilla to plain yogurt smoothies and oatmeal.

Limit Alcohol

Ginni, fifty-one, a university researcher in Michigan, was never much of a drinker, but she used to be able to have two glasses of wine without paying too steep a price. "Now if I have just one glass of wine, I wake up at two a.m. and can't get back to sleep. My skin looks puffier the next day and I feel awful. It's confusing because I weigh the same and I always have something to eat when I drink, so I am not sure why this happens."

There is a biological explanation for what Ginni is experiencing. As you get older, your metabolism slows, causing the sugar in alcohol to stay in your body longer. This is compounded by the loss of lean muscle mass, which is largely responsible for absorbing glucose.

There's mixed evidence that suggests one glass of red wine per day may reduce the risk for cardiovascular disease, but more generally we know that alcohol isn't good for your health. Even small amounts can increase your risk of seven types of cancer, including breast cancer, head and neck cancers, colon cancer, and liver cancer. Researchers surmise that this is due to alcohol's potential to harm DNA as well as its ability to break down certain nutrients that reduce cancer risk, including vitamins C and D, folate, and carotenoids.

I recommend limiting consumption to no more than three glasses of wine (or the equivalent) a week. Along with its extra calories, alcohol can disrupt sleep, which is the last thing you need, and because it dilates blood vessels, it may make hot flashes worse.

Don't Skimp on Sleep

Sleep is one of the first things to suffer during perimenopause and menopause. We've seen how this can raise your risk for several illnesses, from heart disease to diabetes. It also increases the risk of weight gain.

When you are tired, there is a tendency to try to compensate for your lack of energy by upping your calorie (and sugar) intake. Plus, the more hours you spend awake, the more opportunities there are for poor food choices.

Lack of sleep affects appetite on a deeper level as well. When you don't get enough rest, your body produces higher levels of ghrelin, a hormone that increases appetite, and lower levels of leptin, which leads to feeling less full. That leaves you primed to eat more. You are also far less likely to work out if you haven't slept, which compounds the problem. Bottom line: when it comes to weight maintenance, make sleep a priority.

HRT and Weight

Throughout the perimenopausal and menopausal transition, the fluctuations of estrogen affect weight and metabolism. This is such a tough problem for women, it's worth drilling into the science a bit.

There are two main types of estrogen receptors (ERs). The first, ERα (estrogen receptor alpha), is found mainly in the uterus, mammary glands, liver, and cardiovascular system. The second, ERβ (estrogen receptor beta), is found in the ovaries, prostate, lung, colon, and central nervous system.

Estrogen helps to maintain and regulate the energy balance in your body through the receptor ERα. When that gets disrupted during menopause, the result can be an increase in appetite, a decrease in metabolism, and insulin resistance.

Here's why: Androgen levels rise when the follicular ovarian reserves of estrogen get depleted. This creates a hormonal imbalance that affects energy homeostasis, your body's ability to balance energy intake (calories) and expenditure (the rate our bodies *burn* those calories). The hormones that signal hunger and satiety get thrown out of whack, making it harder to manage appetite. As we've seen, loss of estrogen also leads to a redistribution of fat, with more adipose fat accumulating in the abdomen. That's kind of a triple whammy.

Correlation of Estrogen Decline and Weight Composition

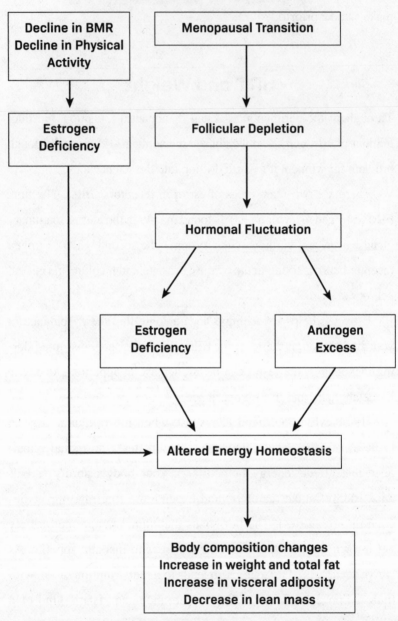

These changes can be mitigated with HRT. Replacing estrogen not only can prevent weight gain but also has been shown to help in weight loss over a three-month period. It has also been found to have a beneficial effect on the insulin response, lipids (including cholesterol), and metabolism.

Plus, it can also help alleviate insomnia, anxiety, and depression, all of which have a propensity to lead to weight gain. To be clear, HRT is not considered and shouldn't be treated as a weight loss drug. It can be a nice benefit, though.

Time–Restricted Eating and Intermittent Fasting

Two approaches that continue to garner attention are time-restricted eating and intermittent fasting. Many people find them helpful, but they are not appropriate for everyone. If you are prone to eating disorders, both should be avoided.

With time-restricted eating (TRE), you set parameters around when you will eat. The time frame is often based around circadian rhythms (your natural sleep/wake cycle) to optimize your body's metabolic response. That means you would plan on eating the bulk of your calories during the front end of the day so that your body can use the fuel as you go about your business. You would then stop eating three hours before bedtime. There is no calorie-counting required. A recent study found that the flexibility of time-restricted eating, which allows you to choose the specific hours you adhere to, may make it easier to stick with.

Intermittent fasting usually involves alternating eating and fasting days, often with five days of eating and then two of fasting. Other approaches include limiting the period of time per day you eat to, say, five hours, so that you are fasting for longer in a single day. Studies have found that while this can lead to weight loss, it is likely due to the reduced calorie intake rather than some magic formula. That said, intermittent fasting has been shown to improve glucose regulation and decrease inflammation.

Emotional Eating Can Be More Tempting than Ever

Dropping hormone levels affect more than just body fat composition. Loss of estrogen can lead to irritability, low energy, anxiety, and stress, all of which make it more tempting to reach for snacks and prepackaged foods that are high in sugar and fat. (It's chips for me.) Depression can lead you to self-medicate with food, by either overeating or opting for unhealthy "comfort foods." Because depression can also make you more sedentary, the effects of the increased caloric intake are compounded by lack of exercise, setting up a vicious cycle. (See Chapter 10, "This Is Your Brain on Menopause.")

Andi, fifty, had always been an avid runner. Her weight never changed until she hit perimenopause, when she quickly gained ten pounds. "I had all these patriarchal standards of what women should look like that were stuck in my head," she says. "It took me a while to come to terms with the changes and accept them as normal. For a while, I was embarrassed to go to the gym because of all the other younger, thinner women there, even though it was something I used to enjoy. I finally got to the point where I realized I was only hurting myself, emotionally and physically. When I exercise now, it's not about how I look but what I can do to ensure I lead an active life as I get older. I never step on the scale anymore. If I can't fit into the pants I wore last year, I'm okay with it."

It's a process—what change isn't?—but when your inner critic starts getting too chatty, you have the authority to shut it down. Imagine how you would talk to a friend. Would you say, *You look awful today*? Never! Then why would you speak to yourself that way?

None of these habits is easy to break, but acknowledging your patterns is the first step. Keisha Henderson has struggled with weight gain throughout menopause, and admits she gives in to emotional eating. She has devised a two-minute pause technique to help get the behavior under control. "I've come to realize that I go for the sweet snacks whenever I'm going through emotional upheavals. Now, when I am about to reach for food, I stop and ask myself, *Am I really hungry?* Often, the answer is no. I may just need a drink of water or I may be angry or disappointed. Just becoming aware of that pattern has helped a lot."

There are other in-the-moment interventions that can help you disrupt the cycle of emotional eating.

- **Keep a mood/food diary.** For one week, write down not just what you eat but what you were feeling when you ate it. Were you stressed? Undergoing relationship turmoil? Seeing the patterns in black and white can help you recognize them and prevent them in the future.

- **Have healthy substitutes within reach.** We tend to grab what is easiest. Keep healthy, satiating foods in the front of your refrigerator and cabinets. Have a stash of them at work. Aim for snacks with protein, which keep you full longer.

- **Brew a cup of herbal tea.** There are many caffeine-free options, including fruit flavors, that can satisfy a craving. Flavored seltzers are also a good bet.

- **Give yourself a manicure.** Not only does painting your nails provide a good distraction, but it's also hard to reach for food when the polish is still wet.

- **Call a friend.** Promise yourself that if you still feel like reaching for the candy bar (or whatever your particular weakness is) after the call, you can indulge. If a call isn't your thing, take a five-minute walk. Chances are good that by the time you are done, the craving will be gone.

Eat Your Way to Better Health

Once you start seeing food as a source of pleasure rather than something to be feared, you can begin to make nutritional adjustments that will lessen the effects of menopause and reduce the risk of chronic diseases for years to come. Here are some of the most effective ways to do that—no deprivation required!

MYTH: Eating fat makes you fat.

FACT: We've all grown fat-phobic when it comes to our diet, but not eating enough healthy fat can lead us to crave unhealthy carbohydrates. For example, choosing 2 percent Greek yogurt as opposed to the fat-free option will be more satisfying and keep you feeling full longer.

Try the Mediterranean Diet

I'm sure you've noticed how many times I've already alluded to the Mediterranean diet throughout this book. The reason: the Mediterranean diet has numerous benefits for health and weight loss.

It has its roots in a study done on health and longevity in seven countries around the Mediterranean basin where traditional dietary habits placed an emphasis on vegetables, fruits, nuts, whole grains, olive oil, beans, fish rich in heart-healthy omega-3s, herbs, and spices. Dairy products were consumed but in lesser amounts. One thing not included: highly processed meats.

While no one eating plan is right for all people, the Mediterranean diet, which is high in protein and fiber, and low in sugar, comes close. One of the beauties of it is that there are no calories to count and an almost infinite number of recipes to adapt it to personal taste.

HEALTHY FOOD SWAPS, MEDITERRANEAN STYLE

These food swaps make sticking to the Mediterranean diet (or a close approximation) easy without sacrificing taste.

FOR	SWAP	TRY
Cooking	Butter	Olive oil
Snacking	Potato chips	Roasted chickpeas
Protein	Beef	Salmon
Sandwich	White bread	Whole wheat pita
Flavor	Salt	Herbs and spices

The Mediterranean diet has specific benefits for menopausal women. Research indicates that it can improve the ratio of lean muscle mass to body fat and may lessen the severity of hot flashes. A cross-sectional study in 481 postmenopausal women showed that a high adherence to the Mediterranean diet helped to reduce waist circumference, including the visceral fat that poses such a health threat. When researchers took a closer look, they found the emphasis on legumes (lentils, chickpeas, and soybeans, for example) in the Mediterranean diet lessons the severity of a range of menopausal symptoms. This makes sense, considering they are rich in isoflavones, compounds that have a chemical structure resembling estrogens and can bind to estrogen receptors. The same study found that this eating plan includes a high intake of omega-3s, which can decrease depression and anxiety, and improve your quality of sleep.

To get started reaping the benefits, aim to include seven to ten portions of fruits and vegetables a day. That may sound like a lot, but a single salad with lettuce, red peppers, tomatoes, and mushrooms already gets you halfway there. Dress your salad with olive oil and you're incorporating another key element. Swap out white rice and pasta for whole grains like brown rice, farro, or quinoa and you have the elements of the Mediterranean diet that you and your family can enjoy.

Boost Your Microbiome and Gut Health

The gut microbiome has been getting a lot of attention recently, and justifiably so. The microbiome lives across your digestive tract and holds an entire universe of microorganisms including bacteria, fungi, viruses, and parasites. That sounds bad, but it's not. Your gut contains 80 percent of your immune cells and helps protect against inflammation, one of the root causes of autoimmune disorders and certain cancers. The more diverse your microbiome is, the better its ability to safeguard you from disease.

The makeup of everyone's microbiome is different and is affected by age, diet, and genetics, as well as environmental factors. And, of course, menopause. (Surprised? Probably not, by this point!) "Estrogen has a protective effect on the gastrointestinal tract," says Stacy Sims, MSC, PhD, an expert in exercise physiology and nutritional science, and one of my go-to gurus. "During perimenopause there's a huge change in the gut microbiome, including a decrease in the number and diversity of the 'good' bugs. This can contribute to changes in how we process insulin and increase the chances of weight gain."

STEPHANIE'S STORY

How I deal with stress eating . . .

In my twenties and thirties, I developed some pretty horrible eating habits. My weight kept climbing, especially as I got into my forties. I have three children, ranging in age from fifteen to twenty-one years old, and I'm a pastor's wife, so the busyness never stops. I didn't make my own weight and health a priority. I'm forty-nine now, and I'm in a season of life when I must start taking better care of myself. I know menopause will make dealing with my weight even harder.

I was intimidated about joining a big gym. I didn't know how to use the equipment and I definitely wasn't going to be one of those people strutting around in a sports bra. I bought a couple of workout outfits that I'm comfortable in, including a big shirt and leggings, and found a trainer who dealt with me as a whole person, from my eating habits to my lifestyle. When she asked me what my goal is, I told her, "I'm not trying to be a size two or size four. I want to be able to walk and not be out of breath. I want to be able to keep up with my family."

She talked to me about the importance of building muscle with strength training, which I'd never done, and tracking my food. The idea that weight training could help me lose weight was totally new to me, but she convinced me that building muscle will not only change my shape and make me stronger, but it will make weight loss more successful. I see her twice a week for full-body strength workouts, and walk three days on my own. It's an investment, and I pay in advance to make sure I go.

One of the surprising things exercise did was help me realize how much I was using food to deal with stress. Working out, and just moving my body, gives me a different outlet and makes me calmer so I'm less likely to grab unhealthy snacks. I used a food diary to track how much of my unhealthy eating was due to emotions. It helped me realize that I reach for cookies whenever I'm particularly tired or stressed.

Sodas are a craving for me, but instead of telling myself I can never have one, I limit it. If I'm at a restaurant, I'll have a glass of water first. Usually after I've had that water, I don't want a Coke anyway. All these little things, like walking, weight training, tracking my food, are gradually adding up.

It's still a process for me. I've lost twenty pounds and I still want to lose thirty more, but I have so much more energy than I previously did. When I have friends who get down on themselves, I always tell them, "Don't mourn whatever size you were in college. Own where you are now and play the long game when it comes to your health."

—Stephanie Carter, 49

Unfortunately, your microbiome's diversity begins to plateau after age forty. The ensuing decline in hormone levels not only reduces this diversity and weakens your immune system, but it can also lead to a more permeable gut barrier, known as "leaky gut." This allows bacteria and toxins to infiltrate the bloodstream, resulting in bloating, and in some cases, inflammatory bowel disease.

An emerging body of research highlights the connection between gut health and brain function. "The gut/brain axis allows bi-directional communication between your brain and microbiome via neurotransmitters," Sims explains.

The moodiness that often comes with menopause? Some of that may be due to changes in your gut. It just so happens that 95 percent of serotonin, the feel-good hormone that helps regulate mood and tame anxiety, is produced in the gut. Fluctuating hormones can impact the communication between the brain and the gut, weakening the delivery of serotonin just when you need it most. "A diminished gut microbiome may even reduce the volume of brain tissue," Sims says. Researchers are currently studying the impact this might have on Parkinson's and Alzheimer's diseases.

Taking the following steps can strengthen your microbiome and protect you from some of these midlife changes.

1. **Increase fiber intake.** Fiber helps maintain gut diversity and provides nourishment for beneficial bacteria. Some examples of fiber-rich foods that benefit the microbiome include whole grains, beans, flax seeds, avocados, apples, and bananas.

2. **Have more fermented foods.** Fermented foods help to increase the amount of good bacteria in your gut. Examples include yogurt with probiotics, kefir, tempeh, sauerkraut, and miso.

3. **Eat the rainbow.** Foods rich in color such as blueberries, cherries, and red cabbage are rich in polyphenols that can help support your gut lining and aid the immune response.

4. **Take a ten-minute walk.** Exercise can help build and maintain a more diverse gut microbiome. A short walk after eating can also speed up digestion and may lower blood sugar levels.

5. **Give your gut a rest.** Giving yourself a break from eating for up to twelve to fourteen hours may help your gut restore and replenish itself. This is easiest for most people to accomplish overnight—for example, if you finish eating at seven p.m. at night, wait until seven the next morning to have breakfast, or even stretch that to nine a.m. if you can.

CHAPTER EIGHT

The Exercise Rx

Don't train to be skinny.
Train to be a #badass.

—DEMI LOVATO

There is no magic pill that will improve every aspect of your physical, psychological, and spiritual health, but one thing comes close: exercise. In fact, I foresee a day when doctors will write a prescription for exercise just as they would for any other course of disease prevention.

Exercise can not only help you retain muscle and aid in weight maintenance, but it can also reduce your risk of heart disease, cancer, and diabetes, and protect your bones from osteoporosis. It can increase your libido and your overall sexual health. (A lesser known but rather nice benefit, right?) But why stop there? Exercise can lower your risk of depression, ease anxiety, improve sleep, give you more energy, improve cognition, and boost your self-confidence. It may even help prevent Alzheimer's disease.

Most of all, exercise just makes you feel good.

While it is important at every stage of life, exercise is especially beneficial for women during perimenopause and menopause. Skeletal muscle mass peaks in our twenties and thirties, after which there is a decline (called sarcopenia) that occurs at a rate of 3 to 8 percent every ten years after the age of thirty. During your forties, fifties, and beyond, the aging process, a sedentary lifestyle, and a decline in estrogen combine to weaken bones and decrease muscle at an accelerated pace. Without intervention, estrogen receptors in your muscles simply aren't getting enough of the hormone they need to thrive.

This raises the risk for osteoporosis, falls, fractures, and overall mortality. On top of that, losing muscle lowers your base metabolic rate (how fast or slow you burn calories), which can lead to weight gain, type 2 diabetes, and other metabolic disorders. According to the American Diabetes Association, exercise can lower your blood sugar levels for up to *twenty-four hours*. Even going for a walk can help your body to absorb glucose from your bloodstream, convert it, and utilize it for fuel.

Your mind also reaps significant benefits from movement. Exercise increases blood flow to the brain and improves executive function. That's what helps you think clearly, switch between tasks, and problem-solve. Even moderate activity may help improve memory by increasing blood flow to the prefrontal cortex, which is responsible for attention. There are more brainy benefits: research shows that exercise improves neuroplasticity, your brain's ability to continue forming new neural connections throughout your life. This can improve learning capacity and response to stress, regardless of age.

The mental health benefits are just as important. There is a reason the former First Lady Michelle Obama once said, "For me, exercise is more than just physical—it's therapeutic." Staying active can help you become more resilient and less anxious, control addictive behaviors (including smoking), and reduce fatigue. Need more encouragement? Just twelve weeks of moderate exercise has been shown to improve vitality, mental health, and quality of life in menopausal women.

I encourage you to begin an exercise program *before* muscle loss accelerates (and fatigue gets the better of you) so that you can lead an active life well into your seventies and eighties. Think about being able to stash a suitcase in the overhead bin, carrying groceries, or having the energy to chase after grandkids in the future. Now is the time to start prepping your body for all your tomorrows.

How Much Exercise Do You Really Need?

Before we get to specific types of exercise, keep in mind that anything you do is better than nothing, and the health benefits begin to accrue as soon as you get off the couch.

Here are some general guidelines to get you started. To improve your overall health, aim for a minimum of 150 minutes of moderate exercise, or 75 to 150 minutes of vigorous aerobic exercise. That works out to about thirty minutes a day, five days a week. Moderate exercise is when you can easily talk (or sing along to your playlist) while you are moving without losing your breath. Cleaning your house, biking on flat ground, or taking a brisk walk all count toward your minutes. Pickleball is the rage for a reason: it's fun, it counts as exercise, and it's a great way to meet people. Vigorous exercise substantially raises your heart rate and breathing. Examples include running, hiking, swimming laps, shoveling snow, or high-impact aerobics.

You don't have to get your thirty minutes all at the same time to reap the benefits. Because sitting for long stretches can be as harmful as smoking, taking short walking breaks throughout the day can be especially beneficial. You've probably heard that 10,000 steps is the best goal for health. Recent studies have shown it may not take that much. Taking even 7,000 steps a day reduces the chance of early death by as much as 70 percent.

Getting Started:
Find Your *Why* and *What*

At a time of life when so much may feel out of your control, choosing to exercise is something you *can* control. Whether you haven't exercised in years, have hit a plateau, or are ready to up your game, being clear about your motivation and having a plan will help you start and stick with it.

Everyone has their own *why*. Your *why* may be brain health, emotional well-being, having more energy, or disease prevention. I can tell you my *why*. One of the first symptoms of perimenopause I experienced was brain fog. I found that exercise makes an enormous difference in mental clarity. I aim for three to four sessions a week. While I used to be a runner, these days I concentrate much more on strength training with heavy weights to build muscle, tone my body, and prevent weight gain. On top of the physical benefits, I love the sense of confidence finishing a challenging session gives me.

After, Rhonda, fifty, was diagnosed with breast cancer, her *why* changed. She was lucky that it was caught early, but treatment required that she go into chemically induced menopause. "It was a lot to handle physically and emotionally," she says. "One of the things I've found most helpful is seeing a personal trainer twice a week. It's definitely an investment in time and money, but I make it a budget priority. Like all women, I was losing muscle and bone mass, my metabolism was dropping, and I was gaining weight around the middle. When I started working out, my goal was to lose ten pounds. I've only lost five so far, but I've gotten stronger and the shape of my body has changed. I fit into clothes I couldn't wear before. What it does for my mood is even more motivating than what it does for my body. Before I go to the gym, I always dread it. I think of everything else I need to do instead: go to the grocery store, do my laundry, get to work. But as soon as I finish a session, I get that dopamine lift. It just feels really good. That's what keeps me going back more than anything."

Terri was motivated by what she wants to accomplish in the future. "When I was younger, I took it for granted that I was always going to be healthy and feel good. The older I got, and especially after having Covid, I realized I couldn't take that for granted. My goal is to see my grandchildren grow up and watch them go out into the world. I knew I couldn't continue as I was, just hoping for the

BUILDING BLOCK

Three Quick Exercise "Snacks"

Sitting for long periods without taking a break can cause an aching back and poor circulation. Breaking that up with even short periods helps to counteract the negative health effect. Try sprinkling these quick fitness snacks throughout the day.

1. **Calf raises:** Standing with your feet planted firmly on the ground, slowly lift your heels until you are balanced on the balls of your feet. Hold for a breath, then lower your heels. Do two sets of twenty to improve ankle strength, balance, and mobility.

2. **Wall push-ups:** Stand facing a wall with your arms bent and your hands placed on the wall at chest level. Keeping your back straight, bend your elbows until your chest grazes the wall, then push back. When you do twenty reps, move on to push-ups on your knees, then toes.

3. **Wall sit:** Stand with your back against a wall with your feet hip-width apart. Keeping your back straight, slide down the wall until your thighs are parallel to the floor. Hold the position for two minutes.

best. Things happen in life—we can get sick, we can fall into ruts—but there are things I can control. Part of that is making a conscious effort to take care of myself. I started walking every day. I'd never tried strength training until a friend at the gym asked me to join her. I was skeptical, but I actually liked it. We go together twice a week and knowing I'm going to meet her there keeps me accountable."

Whatever your personal motivation, keeping your long-term goal in mind can help you prioritize exercise when life pulls you in a million directions. Don't leave it to chance; schedule your workout sessions (even morning walks) ahead of time and enter them into your calendar as you would any appointment. Find a fitness buddy if you can. Remember that it takes ten weeks for something to become a habit. If you miss a day (or even a week), don't beat yourself up or use it as an excuse to give up. Chalk it up to being human and start again. Progress comes from consistency, not perfection.

After choosing your *why,* start thinking about your *what.* There are more workout options than ever, from free online videos to personal trainers to classes at your local Y or boutique fitness center. If you are just starting out, recovering from an injury, or dealing with physical impairments, the fitness trainer Hailey Babcock recommends meeting with a trainer or physical therapist who can provide guidance about proper form, as well as the best activities to preclude future injuries and prevent current conditions, such as tendonitis, from getting worse. Yes, it's an investment, but the payoff in health and safety is worth it if you can afford it.

No matter what activity you choose, diving in too hard, too fast will likely lead to physical and psychological burnout. Plan on a slow,

Eat Your Way to a Better Workout

What and when you eat has a big impact on how you exercise and the results you get. Restricting calories too much becomes a downward spiral where you get tired and don't have the energy to get the results you want. Don't be afraid to fuel up. Stacy Sims recommends eating protein throughout the day to get the most out of a workout. Have a look at a sample of a day's eating for someone who exercises first thing in the morning:

- **Pre-workout:** Half a banana (which has the healthy carbs you need for fuel) and a cold brew coffee with a scoop of protein powder and almond milk or oat milk.

- **Post-workout breakfast:** 2 percent Greek yogurt with some berries and a sprinkle of walnuts or chia seeds.

- **Late-morning snack:** An apple with almond butter, hard-boiled eggs, or some other kind of protein.

- **Lunch:** A big salad with some berries, apples, nuts, or beans (rich in complex carbs) with a serving of protein. (The protein should be the size of the palm of your hand.)

- **Late-afternoon snack:** A handful of nuts or a stick of cheese. If you are working from home, some celery or carrots with hummus is also a good way to go.

- **Dinner:** Stir-fried veggies with brown rice and some lean protein (chicken, fish, tofu). After dinner, stop eating. If you are hungry, try herbal tea or a glass of hot oat or almond milk to cut cravings.

steady course, and always check with your doctor before engaging in any new form of exercise to rule out any underlying health conditions.

Mix It Up

Finding a form of exercise you love, whether it's running, a dance class, barre, or weight machines at the gym will enhance your chances of sticking with it. That might require you to try a few different things, and step outside your comfort zone. No one exercise mode can do it all, and you will get the best results if you mix things up. That will also help you avoid an exercise plateau by challenging your muscles and your brain to reengage.

Cardio is great for your heart, weight training is a must for building muscle and improving bone density, yoga and tai chi help with flexibility, balance, and emotional well-being. That doesn't mean you have to do *everything*, but I do recommend that you balance cardio with at least two strength-training sessions a week. Combining these activities not only improves your physical well-being, but also has been shown to improve your memory more than aerobic exercise alone. When it comes to dealing with brain fog, that's something to keep in mind.

The Importance of Weight Training

Let's get one misconception out of the way: Working out with weights will not bulk you up. Most women don't have enough testosterone for that to happen. Plus, building superhero muscles takes a huge amount of time and *extremely* heavy lifting. What strength training *will* do is give you definition, stave off muscle loss, and improve your overall health. While you may be familiar with the mood-boosting endorphins you get from cardio, studies show that strength training can also significantly reduce depression and improve body image in midlife women as well. It may even help regulate hormone levels and lessen the impact of hot flashes.

When many of us were younger, it was all cardio, all the time. If you did any strength training, it was only with two-pound weights. That was certainly true for me. In college and throughout my twenties, running was my main form of exercise, but as I hit my forties, I began to get a little flabby and my skin was starting to get lax. When I added weight training, using increasingly heavier weights, and ate more protein, my strength increased markedly and my whole body got more toned.

Ideally, you should strength train two to three times a week. "One hour per session is ideal, but if you only have thirty minutes, you can still get a good workout, especially if you do it twice a week," Babcock says. "I recommend doing full-body workouts each session rather than concentrating on legs one day and upper body the next. That way you're hitting all your muscles twice."

To get the best results, you want to use the heaviest weights you can while still practicing good form. The goal is to fatigue the muscle, which improves endurance, increases calorie burn, and recruits the low-twitch and fast-twitch muscle fibers that help overall muscle growth. Lifting heavier weights is particularly important during perimenopause and menopause because it is more effective at increasing bone density, strengthening the connective tissue around bones, and preventing osteoporosis. Because muscles use more glucose, building them up with heavier weights will also help speed your metabolism.

"Heavy" means something different to everyone. One way to find your "heavy" is to start with a weight that fatigues your muscles after six to ten reps of a specific exercise (say, biceps curls). Map out a progressive system that makes each workout a little bit harder than the week before to continually challenge your muscles. Once you can comfortably do two sets of ten repetitions, increase the weight by a small amount and work up to doing the same number of reps with the new weight. Then increase the weight again.

"In the beginning, you will be able to go up in weight pretty quickly," Babcock says. "You may start with five-pound free weights doing biceps curls, and find within a few weeks, you can do the same number of reps with eight-pound weights. After that initial period, building muscle is a slow process, but you should start seeing results in eight to twelve weeks."

You don't need weights or even a gym to improve lower body strength. Squats and lunges work your quadriceps (front of thighs), hamstrings, butt, calves, abductors (inner thigh muscles), core, and lower back. To practice squats, stand with your feet shoulder width apart. Keeping your chest up and shoulders back, bend from the knees as if sitting down in a chair. Aim to get your thighs parallel to the floor before rising. For lunges, start with your feet hip width apart, then take a large step forward with one foot, lowering both knees as close to parallel to the ground as possible. Return to starting position and repeat with the other foot. To begin, do each exercise ten times, then add to the number of reps as you make progress.

One easy way to test your lower body strength and track your progress is the "Sit-to-Stand" test. Use a chair with a seat approximately seventeen inches from the ground. (Make sure the floor is flat.) Starting from a seating position with your arms crossed in front of your chest, see how long it takes you do five sit-to-stand full cycles. A normal range for people forty to fifty-nine is about fifteen repetitions in thirty seconds. (Of course, use your hands if you feel unsteady.)

Don't use your scale to judge your progress. Muscle weighs more than fat, so the number may not budge. How your clothes fit will be a better way to understand how your body composition is changing.

Getting Started with Weight Training

Gyms and your local Y can be great places to meet trainers, make friends, and get access to equipment that you might not have at home. To get the benefits, though, you have to step inside. "The number one reason women in this stage of life aren't going to a gym is intimidation," Babcock says. "I get it. I'm an experienced trainer, I'm fit, and it happens to me, too. I was recently on a business trip and went to a big gym in Las Vegas. Every dude in there was dominating the dumbbells and the benches. I teach exercise routines all day and I still got turned off." Babcock has these tips to get over the intimidation factor of going to a gym.

- **Ask for a tour.** Before you join any gym, including the Y, ask for a tour to get a sense of the vibe. While you are there, ask if someone can spend thirty minutes showing you the equipment. If they are not willing to do that, keep looking. It's also a good idea to visit at the time you will normally be going so you can get a sense of the capacity.

- **Avoid peak hours.** If you can, schedule your gym time when the floor will be less crowded. You will have more time to learn each machine while you gain confidence.

- **Watch video demos of equipment.** It can be confusing to understand how a new piece of equipment works. You can find many examples from certified trainers on YouTube that will give you a better idea of how the machine operates before you go.

- **Check out the class schedule.** If you plan on taking classes, ask to see the lineup to ensure a wide variety of choices and confirm that the ones you are interested in fit with your schedule.

- **Get a fitness buddy.** Having an exercise partner can keep you accountable. If you have a friend to sign up and go with, great. If not, why not go up to someone you see at the gym and start a conversation? They may be looking for a motivation booster as well.

- **Meet with a trainer.** If you can afford it, a personal trainer who understands your body and your goals can be a worthwhile investment. Even if you just meet with them a handful of times, they can show you proper form and set up a program that you can follow on your own.

HIIT It Up

High-intensity interval training (HIIT) is one of the most effective and time-efficient ways to improve heart health and stimulate stem cell proliferation, which helps with tissue repair and wound healing and promotes healthy aging. During a HIIT workout, you vary short bursts of intense effort with recovery periods. By "intense" I mean something you can sustain only for a very brief amount of time. It should be difficult to hold a conversation. Let's use running as an example. A beginning HIIT plan could consist of two minutes of light jogging or speed walking, followed by thirty seconds of all-out running, repeating the cycle for twenty minutes. As you progress, you can gradually change the ratio of exertion to recovery; say, one minute of light jogging to one minute of all-out running. The approach can be adapted to virtually any form of cardio exercise: a stationary bike, an elliptical trainer, a stair climber, or a rowing machine. At home, you can try HIIT using intervals of jumping jacks or running in place with slower periods of walking or simply stepping sideways for recovery.

HIIT workouts are short on time but long on benefits, including improving your endurance, speeding up metabolism, and lowering your fat to muscle mass ratio. They have even been shown to decrease the risk for heart disease, breast cancer, metabolic syndrome, and arthritis. Because HIIT workouts are designed to be intense, they can be hard on your body if done too frequently. Twice a week for twenty minutes is a good goal.

The Power of Plyometrics

Plyometrics are essentially quick, dynamic bursts of movement that recruit muscles for a short amount of time. It involves a rapid stretch (eccentric contraction) of a muscle, immediately followed by a powerful contraction (concentric contraction). Jumping is a perfect example. Incorporating plyometrics into your workouts can help to increase strength and speed, and is effective for preventing osteoporosis. "The eccentric movement involved (say, when you are crouching to jump) helps your muscles store energy, and the concentric movement when you contract the muscles releases energy," Sims says. "This can lead to better overall muscle quality and speed up your metabolism." Warm up your muscles before starting, and if you are jumping, land on soft knees to protect your joints.

You can get the benefit of plyometrics without jumping. "Stand facing a wall with your hand pressed against it, elbows bent. Push yourself away from the wall with a quick movement until your hands leave the surface, then return to the starting position. This is essentially a wall push-up where you grab some air," Sims says.

Soothe Your Mind, Strengthen Your Body: Yoga and Tai Chi

Mind-body workouts, including yoga and tai chi, can reduce the frequency and intensity of hot flashes and help you sleep better. Both can ease muscle and joint pain, strengthen your pelvic floor, and lead to better balance, posture, and flexibility.

"Yoga is so much more than a physical practice," says my friend Gabrielle Espinosa, a yoga instructor who specializes in movement for women going through menopause. "You engage your muscles, build strength, and burn calories, but it is really a practice for helping you tune in to inner awareness." It is great for helping you manage stress, which is one of the biggest drivers of menopausal symptoms including insomnia and brain fog. It can lessen the chances of depression and may even help prevent dementia. And the benefits can begin after just twelve weeks.

As with all forms of exercise, it is best to start slowly and learn proper form to avoid injuries. Most yoga studios, gyms, and Ys have beginner classes. Talk to the teacher ahead of time, tell them that you are new to yoga, and don't be shy about sharing any physical limitations you might have. There are also free videos online that can demonstrate proper form. Here are some of the most common types of yoga:

- **Hatha:** This practice includes slow, progressive movement and is a great place to start.

- **Vinyasa:** You will be guided through flowing poses at a slightly faster pace, matching your breath to each pose.

- **Bikram:** Practiced in a heated room, an instructor will guide you through twenty-six poses. Be prepared to sweat. A lot.

KEISHA'S STORY

I'm FINALLY learning to feel at home in my body.

My first real yoga experience didn't happen until the fifth time I went to class. It was at the end where you lay down in savasana. Suddenly, I started crying. I jumped off my mat, thinking, *What is this voodoo stuff?* It took me a while to realize yoga was the only place where I took a deep breath. The tears were such a release. I kept going back because there was something there I needed.

Combining breath and body work in yoga helps me feel at home in my body. I went from a B to a D cup when I first gained weight. I've had to learn to navigate in this new body and accept it as this beautiful thing. There's just more of me to love.

Yoga also helps me shift out of ruminating thoughts. Any time I am moving and meditating at the same time, it just breaks the negativity loop. I know so many women who think, *Oh, I could never be a yogi.* Sometimes those self-limiting beliefs are deeply ingrained, but you just have to start with some acceptance of where you are now and trust in the practice. It's never too late to start.

—Keisha Henderson, 52

- **Restorative:** Designed to create a state of calm, you will engage in a series of passive poses (as in lying down) and meditation.

Tai chi, which is rooted in martial arts, marries breath to slow, gentle movements designed to move chi, or energy, throughout your body. While you may think of it as an "old" person's exercise, it's increasingly popular with women in their forties and fifties. The ancient form of exercise improves balance and bone density, and can enhance cognitive function.

Bolster Your Balance

After the age of thirty or thirty-five, we start to lose our balance, which is the biggest risk factor in falls, one of the leading causes of mortality later in life. Want a quick litmus test? People who are unable to stand on one leg for ten seconds in midlife have almost double the risk of premature death. That is ten seconds worth investing in.

While strength training, yoga, and tai chi can all help with balance, Babcock recommends adding targeted exercises into your routine as well. "One easy way to improve balance is to grab a can of soup, a bottle of water, or a two-pound or three-pound weight, and stand on one leg. With the other slightly bent at the knee, pass the weight back and forth. Then repeat the exercise, changing legs. Doing this barefoot has the added benefit of working your ankle and foot stabilizers, which are often overlooked in exercise programs." Extra points if you can do it with your eyes closed. I practice balancing on one leg at a time while brushing my teeth, which my kids find very amusing.

CHAPTER NINE

Thin Skin, Thinner Hair

I can't think of any better
representation of beauty than someone
who is unafraid to be herself.

—EMMA STONE

Dry, irritated skin. Bruises. Breakouts. Too much hair where you don't want it (your face). Too little hair where you *do* want it (your head). These are just some of the changes fluctuating hormone levels can unleash on your appearance.

Estrogen spurs the growth of collagen, a protein that helps support skin, muscle, and bones. It is essentially the scaffolding that holds everything up. During the first five years of menopause, though, your skin loses about 30 percent of its collagen. "After that, the decline is more gradual," says the New York dermatologist Dendy Engelman, MD. "Women will lose about ten percent of their collagen every year for the next twenty years."

As collagen declines, your skin becomes drier and thinner, making it prone to wrinkling and sagging. Skin becomes more translucent. Bruises become more apparent, as do dark circles under your eyes, regardless of how much melanin you have. The skin barrier—the outer layer that protects against irritants, pollution, and loss of moisture—weakens as adhesions between the skin cells become less tight. "Women come to me confused when the same product that they have loved for years suddenly irritates their skin," Dr. Engelman says. "Because menopause weakens the skin barrier, the same products penetrate at a different level and can cause a number of reactions, from itchiness and irritation to red blotches." Even your nails can be affected, becoming drier, more brittle, and prone to breaking.

Changing hormone levels also affect the output of sebum (the somewhat oily product of the sebaceous glands). For some women, a decrease in sebum can cause further dryness, redness, and inflammation. In other cases, sebum can clog pores, leading to breakouts.

Ginni, fifty-one, was unprepared for what happened when she entered menopause, despite having read extensively about it. "The changes I saw in the mirror didn't help my already sinking confidence," she says. "My skin got drier and looser, and my hair started thinning. The temples on the side of my face were bare, which made me very self-conscious." Ginni's first step was to go on an estrogen patch. "That helped my mood, which was the most important thing, but it also made my skin look a little plumper." Next, she went to a dermatologist, who prescribed minoxidil for her thinning hair. "Within five months, I started to see a difference," she says. "When

I pull my hair up for yoga, I don't see scalp anymore. It's not going to turn me into Rapunzel, but it is keeping the hair loss from getting worse. Combining HRT, richer moisturizers, and being diligent about minoxidil makes me feel like I'm slowing the process down instead of going into freefall."

Moisturize, Moisturize, and Moisturize More

Moisturizing the skin on your face and body will not only help it look better, but can also prevent the itchiness and flaking that menopause can bring. You will probably need to switch to richer moisturizer than you used when you were younger to counteract these changes. Dr. Engelman suggests looking for moisturizers with ceramides, which help to maintain the skin barrier and retain moisture. "Ceramides are fatty acids that make up approximately forty percent of your skin," she explains. "As estrogen levels drop, ceramide production decreases. That means we're not making these new proteins that create the mortar between the skin cells. You replenish this "glue" between cells with products that contain ceramides and mimic the skin barrier." Hyaluronic acid, a natural lubricant your body produces, is another great ingredient to look for in oils and moisturizers. There are a number of face and body products at all price points that fit the bill. Applying moisturizer while your skin is still damp can help it retain moisture, and eating a diet that includes healthy fats including nuts, olive oil, and oily fish can also help your skin.

Applying oil and thick hand creams, along with wearing gloves both outside and while doing dishes, can help protect the skin on your hands and your nails.

Wash This Way

As your skin thins and the skin barrier weakens, you need to treat it more carefully. Avoid harsh soaps and cleansers, including those containing hydroxy acids, which can be too harsh on thinner skin. Because fragrance can also cause dryness and allergic reactions, look for gentle, fragrance-free soaps and cleansers. It might sound counterintuitive, but oil-based cleansers and balms can do a good job of lifting off makeup without stripping the skin barrier.

Exfoliating can remove debris, dead skin cells, and flakiness, and help moisturizers seep in, but you need to be careful. Avoid physical exfoliants, in the form of either a rough washcloth (which can also harbor bacteria if not washed after each use) or grainy scrubs. Instead, exfoliate once a week with a mild chemical exfoliant such as AHA acid, and follow with a rich moisturizer.

Rebuild Collagen

Vitamin A derivatives, known as retinoids, are the gold standard when it comes to rebuilding collagen to improve fine lines, wrinkles, and pigmentation, as well as to spur cell turnover. They work by promoting the shedding of old, damaged skin cells and stimulating the growth of new, healthier cells. This process helps to keep the skin's

MYTH: Drinking a Lot of Water Will Help My Skin Stay Hydrated

FACT: Drinking water is excellent for virtually every aspect of your health, but unless you are experiencing severe dehydration, it won't help your skin stay hydrated or prevent wrinkles. "There's not a direct one-to-one correlation of oral hydration and skin hydration," Dr. Engelman says. "Skin hydration is a function of sebaceous gland density and sebaceous gland activity, which produce sebum, an oily substance that protects and moisturizes skin, and can fluctuate depending on hormone levels." Applying a moisturizer is a much better way to hydrate skin. But drink up anyway. Water is still good for you.

surface smooth and reduces clogged pores. Retinoids can also help ward off acne by preventing the accumulation of dead skin cells and oil in hair follicles. Retinoids are available in a range of formulations and price points, from prescription-strength Retin-A (sold generically as tretinoin) to milder over-the-counter retinols.

Because light and air can reduce the effectiveness of retinoids, it is best to use them at night. This aligns with skin's natural circadian rhythm, supporting the product's effectiveness in promoting cell turnover and collagen synthesis. The immediate effect is often flaking as your skin sheds its top layer. One way to counteract the irritation is to

Five Skincare Ingredients to Look For

You don't have to spend a fortune to put together an effective skincare routine. These days, there are products at all price points, from drugstore options to luxe lines, that can make a real difference. Dr. Engelman suggests these five ingredients to look for, along with retinoids and vitamin C. Do a skin patch test of any new product by putting a dab of it on your inner arm and waiting twenty-four hours to rule out an allergic reaction.

- **Hyaluronic acid (HA):** HA is a naturally occurring substance found throughout your body that helps joints stay lubricated. It is exceptionally good at retaining moisture, which can help skin stay flexible and prevents wrinkles. Found in serums and moisturizers, it is safe for most skin types.

- **Peptides:** Polypeptides are fragments of proteins that help rebuild collagen, boosting skin's ability to retain moisture. Peptides contain antioxidants, which can help fight inflammation, protect the skin barrier, and reduce the appearance of wrinkles. Look for peptides in serums and moisturizers.

- **Ceramides:** These fatty acids contain lipids that help maintain the skin barrier by locking in moisture and blocking out pollutants and other irritants, to make skin look moist and plumper. Ceramides are also effective in treating eczema.

- **Niacinamide:** A form of vitamin B3, niacinamide is touted for its skin-brightening ability, can reduce redness, and can be useful in combating acne. It can be applied once a day after your moisturizer. Because those with sensitive skin may experience a slight tingling or burning sensation, do a patch test for a few days first.

- **SPF:** Using SPF every day, rain or shine, cloudy or bright, is the most important step you can take to prevent skin cancer and premature aging.

start slowly, using your chosen formula every other night as your skin adjusts. You can buffer the effects by applying a moisturizer before and after you apply Retin-A. Dr. Engelman recommends beginning with a formula that has a lower percentage of retinol and building up to greater strengths. Use a pea-size amount and spread it evenly across your face. As you continue to use retinoids, skin cells will replicate and the collagen will slowly rebuild, leaving you with stronger, clearer, and more robust skin. It can take a few months to see the full effect, so be patient.

All retinoids make skin more sensitive to sun, regardless of your ethnicity or complexion, so you must be extra careful to use a sunscreen with a strong SPF every day, rain or shine. Your skin may also be more sensitive to active ingredients in other skin products, so stick to rich, mild moisturizers. Retinoids can be effective at treating the under-eye area, but because the skin is thinner there, look for creams that are ophthalmology-tested and made specifically for this.

Get Your Vitamin C

Vitamin C is another ingredient with strong scientific research that backs up its ability to fight the damage caused by free radicals, including photoaging and hyperpigmentation, and calm the effects of inflammation. Most topical solutions, whether serums or moisturizers, contain L-ascorbic acid, the active form of the vitamin C. Formulations vary in strength, usually ranging from 5 to 20 percent. Formulas with a higher percentage may be more effective, but they can also sting and cause irritation. As with Retin-A, start at the lower end and see how your skin reacts. Because vitamin C is an unstable molecule, it loses its power when exposed to light, so look for dark packaging and keep it away from the sun. It is safe to use vitamin C with other skincare products, but Dr. Engelman recommends using it in the morning, followed by sunscreen.

Breakouts? Seriously?

Approximately 25 percent of women in their forties experience breakouts not unlike those that occur in puberty. In this case, it is usually due to hormonal imbalances as estrogen decreases and testosterone levels fluctuate. It can be particularly frustrating if you have dry skin on your cheeks and pimples on your nose or jawline. It will take a two-pronged attack that includes moisturizing the dry areas of your face and spot treatment for breakouts.

While adult acne may remind you of your teen years, you should treat it differently from what you did when you were younger. "Your skin is thinner and probably too sensitive for harsh spot treatments," Dr. Engelman says. "Retinoids, whether over-the-counter or prescription strength, can be helpful. If the problem persists, your dermatologist may prescribe metronidazole, a topical antibiotic used to treat adult acne and rosacea."

In-Office Procedures That Build Collagen

In-office procedures done by a licensed dermatologist can definitely make a difference in combating signs of skin aging, but there is no denying they are a luxury. Depending on where you live, these treatments can run from a few hundred dollars to thousands. If you have the time and money to invest, Dr. Engelman suggests these two procedures to help build collagen. (Botox and fillers can smooth wrinkles if that's the way you want to go, but they don't build collagen.)

- **Non-ablative Fraxel lasers:** There are a number of Fraxel laser options that vary in depth of skin penetration, recovery time, and cost, but the concept behind them remains the same. Lasers focus tiny beams of heat into the epidermis without breaking the skin surface. This stimulates a wound-healing response that increases collagen production, resulting in tighter, clearer skin. Skin is numbed before the treatment, which takes about twenty minutes and feels like tiny pinpricks. Non-ablative options are less aggressive and require less recovery time; skin will be red and can be flaky for a couple of days. In the right hands, lasers can also be used on the neck and eyelids, where skin is the thinnest and tends to show aging first. If you are Black, be sure to see a dermatologist experienced in treating darker skin tones, as too high a frequency can result in permanent skin lightening.

- **Microneedling with radio frequency:** Tiny needles are used to transmit the heat from radio frequency beneath the skin surface to create micro-wounds without causing external harm. As the internal layers heal, collagen and elastin forms, which results in fewer lines and more resilient skin. With this technique, there is no risk of inflammatory hyperpigmentation, which makes it appropriate for all skin types and colors.

Too Much Hair
Where You Don't Want It . . .

A decrease in estrogen and an increase in androgens can cause unwanted hair growth on the chin, jaw, or above the lip. "So many women suddenly find a long white hair and think, 'Oh my God, how long has that been there? Did everyone see it?'" Dr. Engelman says. Part of the problem is that because white hairs are harder to spot, you tend not to see them until they are quite long. "I have a contract with my best friends," Stacy, fifty-one, says. "If any of us ends up in a coma, we promise to go over and pluck out their chin hairs while their partner is out of the room."

Options for dealing with unwanted facial hair include electrolysis, shaving, plucking, or waxing. Laser is a safe option for all skin colors and types and will keep hair away for months, or even years. It can be costly, but it may not take long if it is a matter of just a few hairs. "If you are considering a laser treatment, I strongly recommend you jump on it as soon as you see the first dark hair. Lasers will not work once hairs turn white," Dr. Engelman cautions.

. . . And Too Little Hair Where You Do

Hair follicles contain estrogen receptors, which is why, when estrogen and progesterone levels dip, many women experience hair thinning and loss. Heat tools and harsh dyes can cause weak hair to break, exacerbating the problem. Declining hormones also cause eyebrows to thin as we age, with some follicles ceasing to produce hair. Latisse, a topical serum that requires a prescription, is FDA approved to treat thin eyelashes, but it may also help regrow brows. It is not recommended for people with glaucoma, macular edema, or eye inflammation. Results are usually seen in four months.

The actress Gabrielle Union opened up to *People* magazine about her menopausal hair loss. "All of it can feel very isolating and you can feel like less of a woman, especially as a Black woman where our hair is our crown. There's literally the CROWN Act[2] and I'm like, uh, my crown looks more like a barrette at this moment," she said. "It was the hot flashes, the night sweats that could happen at any time of day, brain fog, mood changes, ongoing sadness, anxiety that felt more like terror, hair loss, and then random weight gain. That's when it really hit home for me."

"Biotin, one of the 'B' vitamins, promotes the production of keratin, a protein needed for strong hair and nails. Some research shows that it may help prevent hair loss, but it is not a miracle drug," Dr. Engelman says. "Unless you are one of the very rare people with a biotin deficiency, the jury is out on its effectiveness. There is a risk of taking too much, which can cause stomach issues. Don't take more than three thousand milligrams per day. It is definitely not a case of 'more is better.'" Instead, she recommends speaking to a board-certified dermatologist as soon as you start to notice hair loss to get ahead of the situation. "They may prescribe topical or oral minoxidil, which enhances hair growth and prevents further loss as long you stay on it," she says.

---

2   The CROWN Act bans employers from discriminating against natural hair styles.

Feed Your Face

Along with topical treatments, foods rich in antioxidants can help skin stay supple and may reduce hair breakage. Red grapes are packed with resveratrol, one of the most powerful antioxidants for skin. Resveratrol can help fight the effects of sun damage, including discoloration and wrinkling, and aid in wound healing, and may even help slow or prevent skin cancer. Plus, it enhances collagen production by activating estrogen receptors in the skin. Another reason to grab a bunch of grapes for dessert: resveratrol is good for heart health.

Vitamin C is not just a stellar ingredient in serums and creams. Foods that are rich in vitamin C increase collagen, the protein that strengthens skin and hair. Beta carotene (found in red peppers, sweet potatoes, and carrots) is converted to vitamin A in your body, which fights the free radicals that lead to skin aging. For a food with (added) benefits: Tomatoes have the skin-saving combo of vitamin C and beta carotene, plus lycopene and lutein, powerful antioxidants that protect your skin against damage from UV rays, including dryness, wrinkling, and discoloration. Fatty fishes such as salmon have omega-3 fatty acids that help fight inflammation, keep your hair healthy and your skin soft, and have even been found to prevent psoriasis. Finally, consider adding soy products into your diet. They contain isoflavones, which mimic the role of estrogen, and have been proven to increase collagen and decrease wrinkles.

CHAPTER TEN

This Is Your Brain on Menopause

Nobody is perfect, so get over the fear
of being or doing everything perfectly.
Besides, perfect is boring.

—JILLIAN MICHAELS

An accountant I know who deals with balance sheets all day suddenly couldn't remember the word "revenue." A detail-oriented marketing executive has to read every memo three times instead of once. Another friend forgets the entire storyline of television shows within a day. None of these women are losing their minds, even though it can feel that way. What they *are* losing is estrogen, which affects the brain wiring responsible for memory and how fast you process information. Combine that with a lack of sleep common in menopause and you have a perfect recipe for brain fog.

"Estrogen is to the brain what fuel is to an engine," says Lisa Mosconi, PhD, associate professor of Neuroscience in Neurology and Radiology at Weill Cornell Medicine. "Estrogen, particularly estradiol, the strongest form, plays a critical role in the brain's health and functionality, earning it the title of the 'master regulator' of women's brain health. When estrogen is in the house, everything works well." She explains the four key roles estrogen plays. It helps protect neural structures and cells from damage and promotes the survival of neurons. It is involved in cognitive processes such as memory, learning, and executive functions. It influences mood and emotional well-being, acting on serotonin and other neurotransmitter systems. And finally, estradiol promotes the growth of new neurons and supports neuroplasticity, including the brain's ability to change and adapt.

"After menopause, the decline of estrogen impacts all of these brain functionalities. It's akin to an orchestra that continues to play but to a markedly different tune," Dr. Mosconi says. "Without the guiding influence of estrogen, the brain's regulatory mechanisms, protective functions, and cognitive processes may be altered, potentially leading to changes in memory, mood, and overall brain health."

Nearly two-thirds of women report cognitive symptoms during perimenopause and menopause, including increased stress, anxiety, brain fog, and memory loss. Carol Mehas, a New York executive, was at the top of her profession when she hit menopause. "I'm very Type A but suddenly I felt completely off my game at work. I couldn't control when hot flashes or brain fog would hit. I have a nice husband and beautiful kids, but everything felt off at home, too. It left me feeling helpless and completely alone."

Mood and memory issues can be frustrating (*What was that word again?*) and scary (*Am I getting early-onset dementia?*), and can have a negative effect on relationships (*Why does everything my partner does suddenly annoy me?*). For many women, the symptoms manifest as a vague sense of flatness or lack of spark; for others, outright anger.

Ren, fifty-one, felt her entire personality change. "If you talked to my kids, my husband, or friends, they would have told you I am even-keeled, patient, kind, and friendly, but as soon as I went into perimenopause, I stopped being the same lighthearted person they knew," she says. "I couldn't stand the sound of my husband's voice. He has this lovely Australian accent, and I told him to stop talking to me. We have a great marriage, but he drove me absolutely bonkers. Everything annoyed me and made me feel uncomfortable."

Drew Barrymore recently described how she experienced hormonal fluctuations on the *Today* show. "You go through an emotional roller coaster, and you don't know what's happening, and there aren't indicators there to help it make sense to you, so you just do whatever it is you can to be calmer so that you will be better for yourself, as well as those around you."

Your Brain Goes through Estrogen Withdrawal

Estrogen receptors in various regions of the brain interact with the neurotransmitters responsible for mood, memory, and cognition. Think of neurotransmitters as little chemical messengers that send signals between nerve cells throughout the body. As hormone levels dip during perimenopause and menopause, these signals weaken and your brain goes through estrogen withdrawal. Three of the neurotransmitters most affected by this include serotonin, dopamine, and norepinephrine.

Serotonin promotes a sense of calm, well-being, and happiness. Low serotonin levels can lead to irritability and anxiety, which, along with making you generally cranky, can disrupt sleep. There are strategies that can help you offset low serotonin. Eight weeks of aerobic exercise has been shown to increase both serotonin and endorphins. The vitamin D you get from spending as little as fifteen minutes in sunlight also boosts serotonin levels. To get the benefit of both, try instituting a walking break in the morning or at lunchtime. (Certain antidepressants are designed to increase serotonin in your brain. We'll get to those in a bit.)

Dopamine, another key neurotransmitter modulated by estrogen, influences the reward and pleasure centers in the brain. When dopamine is low, it not only creates depressive moods, but also impacts motivation, concentration, and energy. Yoga, meditation, and walking may all increase dopamine. Eating foods with magnesium and tyrosine, an amino acid, can boost dopamine production. Foods to try include chicken, almonds, apples, avocados, bananas, beets, chocolate, leafy green vegetables, and green tea.

Estrogen also impacts norepinephrine, the neurotransmitter that regulates the fight-or-flight response, and can increase alertness. Imbalances can raise blood pressure, and cause anxiety and panic. This is why some women get panic attacks during menopause. Exercise and meditation can help to regulate norepinephrine.

There's a reason I keep mentioning meditation. Mindfulness is one of the most powerful tools to improve overall mood and brain health. Certain techniques and behaviors like deep breathing and intentional focus (consciously directing your attention to what is happening in the present moment to minimize distractions) decrease stress, anxiety, irritability, and rumination. Meditation can also reduce the discomfort of hot flashes and improve sleep quality, both of which affect your mental state.

Diet can also play a role. Snacking on foods high in salt, sugar, and oil can feel like a temporary fix if you are feeling low, but you are bound to crash soon after and then crave more, which has a detrimental effect on both mood and weight. Melissa Mondala, MD, an expert in women's nutrition, suggests incorporating foods that are proven to have a positive effect on mood into your diet. "Foods high in omega-3 and healthy fats may help to strengthen membranes in the brain and improve the flow of neurotransmitters," she says. "They are also high in tryptophan and tyrosine, which are precursors to serotonin and dopamine, the happy hormones that make us feel good." Look for sesame and pumpkin seeds, flax seeds, and pistachio nuts for a mood-boosting snack.

HRT and Brain Health

Along with exercise, meditation, a diet rich in fiber and antioxidants, and getting enough sleep, hormone replacement therapy can help to counter the effects of the loss of estrogen on mood and cognition, especially when you get a jump start and begin HRT during perimenopause.

Foods That Improve Your Mood

Foods high in B vitamins and healthy fats can help to strengthen membranes in the brain, improve the flow of neurotransmitters, reduce mood swings, and support neurotransmitters. Dr. Mondala suggests incorporating almonds, walnuts, and pecans into your diet. Be careful not to overindulge, though, as they can be high in calories. Here are her suggestions for incorporating some other feel-food foods into your diet:

- Mix ground flax seeds into a smoothie, oatmeal, or pancakes. Sprinkle them onto brown rice or quinoa.

- Make chia seed pudding by mixing the seeds with soy or almond milk and adding your favorite berries for added antioxidants.

- Toss sesame seeds on roasted vegetables and salads.

- Roast pumpkin seeds and add them to your salad instead of croutons.

"There is a 'critical window' theory that suggests the most beneficial time to start HRT for brain health is from perimenopause to the onset of menopause or shortly thereafter," Dr. Mosconi says. "Starting HRT more than ten years after menopause or after the age of sixty may not provide the same potential benefits and could come with some increased health risks, depending on formulation and route of administration."

The short-term benefits of HRT include alleviating hot flashes, night sweats, mild depression due to perimenopause, and sleep disturbances, all of which can affect cognitive function, brain fog, and quality of life. "There is ongoing research into whether HRT can provide long-term neuroprotective effects, potentially reducing the risk of neurodegenerative diseases like Alzheimer's," Dr. Mosconi adds. "The benefits seem to depend on the timing of initiation. Here, too, the 'critical window' hypothesis suggests starting HRT around the time of the onset of menopause may be more beneficial. Lower levels of estrogen in the postmenopausal phase have been associated with an increased plaque buildup that contributes to Alzheimer's. However, the data is mixed, and HRT's role in reducing the incidence of neurodegenerative diseases is still under investigation."

Depression

Approximately 20 percent of women experience some degree of depression during menopause. That's alarming, but in some ways not surprising. Hormones play a big role, but they aren't the only cause. There are other external factors to consider.

Society continues to bombard us with outdated notions of women and aging. Representation across media of older women, especially those who choose to age naturally, continues to lag, while youth is held up as the paradigm. On the job front, it can be a time when women struggle to re-enter the workforce, feel stuck in their careers, or find themselves reporting to people younger than them. Family stress is often at its height as we get sandwiched between taking care of our kids and our elders. A lack of social support, as well as education level, social demographic, and cultural experiences that impact different races and ethnicities, can all contribute to the risk for depression. These factors go a long way to explain why depression is more common among Black and Hispanic women. In fact, Black Americans are twice as likely as white Americans to experience depression.

These societal factors along with a woman's menopausal status should be taken into account when health care providers screen for depression and consider treatment options. Having a full picture of the *entire* scope of a woman's experience may allow for earlier intervention with complementary and alternative modalities such as cognitive behavioral therapy (CBT), mindfulness, acupuncture, yoga, and tai chi, all of which can have a beneficial effect on the mood and behavioral changes women go through during menopause.

Women often ask me how they can tell whether their depression is due to menopause or life circumstances. The answer could be all of the above. The deeper point is, it may not matter. While HRT and, if necessary, antidepressants and/or therapy can in many cases be beneficial, the proactive lifestyle steps you can take to deal with stress, anxiety, or depression are the same regardless of the cause.

While I always advocate for a lifestyle approach to physical and mental health, depression and anxiety can be serious medical conditions and need to be treated as such. If you have a history of depression or have overwhelming feelings of sadness that last for more than two weeks or are interfering with your ability to function, it is important to seek professional help. If you don't have a therapist, ask your general practitioner for a recommendation. If you are in immediate distress, reach out to the suicide and crisis hotline at 988.

Your doctor may recommend antidepressants and/or anti-anxiety drugs. Determining the right medication, the dose, and how long to take them is a complex process that varies from person to person. There are a range of drugs that operate differently. It often takes a period of trial and error to find out what works for you. The medications all come with potential side effects and drug interactions, though they can be taken with HRT.

The two most common classes of antidepressants are serotonin-norepinephrine reuptake inhibitors (SNRIs) and selective serotonin reuptake inhibitors (SSRIs). SSRIs are designed to increase the amount of serotonin available. SNRIs affect both serotonin and norepinephrine levels.

It can take four to six weeks to feel the full effect once you start taking antidepressants. Often the best results come when they are combined with talk therapy. Always work with a doctor if you decide to stop. They will help you taper off slowly, which is usually safer. (See Chapter 4, "The ABCs of HRT," for more specific information on antidepressants, including brand names.)

Brain Fog and Memory Loss

Desiree Jordan, an interior designer, didn't just have trouble remembering names; she could barely focus on what she was doing from one minute to the next. "I had so much trouble remembering what people told me five minutes ago that I began to worry I was getting early-onset Alzheimer's," she says. "I couldn't focus my attention on anything long enough to get tasks done. I had a new job, which was hard enough, and this just made it worse." She found HRT helped.

The fear that brain fog is a sign of dementia is one I hear nearly every day. Let me reassure you: not being able to remember a word does not mean you have early-onset Alzheimer's. One more note of reassurance: Brain fog and memory lapses eventually plateau. The influence of menopausal symptoms on long-term Alzheimer's risk is still being investigated, but what we do know is that, while your genetic blueprint matters, a healthy lifestyle that includes diet, exercise, and maintaining social connections can help to mitigate the effects of your DNA.

Hormonal changes can make existing cognitive conditions, including ADD and ADHD, more intense during perimenopause and menopause. Terri, a retail manager in Kentucky, was diagnosed with ADD years ago. "My symptoms got ten times worse once I went into perimenopause. I have had ADD for years and know how to make accommodations, but the same techniques stopped working. My brain would go to twenty zillion different places. I had to find new ways of handling it. I make lists for everything. Even things as simple as bringing my daughter to voice lessons won't happen if it isn't in my planner. Aside from writing everything down, the one thing I discovered that really helps is yoga. I had never done it before, but I found a community at one particular studio that gave me the incentive to keep going. It took about six months for it to become a habit, but now I won't miss it. It helps tame that scattered feeling and lets me feel more in control, even after I leave class."

Lower Your Risk of Alzheimer's Disease

People who adhered to four to five of the following healthy behaviors have a 60 percent lower risk of Alzheimer's disease. These same steps lower your risk for a number of other diseases including cardiovascular disease, diabetes, and some cancers.

- **At least 150 minutes per week of moderate- to vigorous-intensity physical activity.** In a longitudinal study of midlife women, high levels of cardiovascular fitness were related to a lower risk of dementia.

- **Not smoking.** Even in people sixty years old and up who have been smoking for decades, quitting will lower your risk of dementia.

- **Light to moderate alcohol consumption.** As we get older, we have a heightened sensitivity to alcohol, making us more susceptible to its effects, including memory loss.

- **Cognitive activities.** Being intellectually engaged may help the brain become more adaptable and compensate for age-related changes. Taking up a new hobby, learning a language, reading, and playing games can all keep your mind fired up.

The MIND Diet

The MIND (Mediterranean-DASH Intervention for Neuro-degenerative Delay) diet is specifically designed to support brain health and reduce the risk of Alzheimer's disease. It focuses on plant-based foods and limits servings of red meat, sweets, cheese, butter/margarine, and fast/fried food, and encourages eating from these healthy food groups:

- Leafy green vegetables, at least six servings per week

- Other vegetables, at least one serving per day

- Berries, at least two servings per week

- Whole grains, at least three servings per day

- Fish, one serving per week

- Poultry, two servings per week

- Beans, three servings per week

- Nuts, five servings per week

- Olive oil

Irritability, Stress, and Anxiety

It is not uncommon for emotions you have kept bottled up for years to erupt during menopause. Because they can seem to come out of the blue, you may not understand why you suddenly feel a burst of rage, anger, or irritability. That can lead to an unfortunate tendency to pile on yourself with thoughts like *I shouldn't be feeling this way.*

Anna, forty-nine, has two teenagers and a busy job. "I'm always a little stressed," she admits, "but it went over the top recently. I was in the car with my fourteen-year-old daughter and she was being cranky. I completely flew off the handle. I was right to get annoyed, but my response was so exaggerated, and I yelled so loudly, it scared us both. Afterward, I realized that wasn't how I have handled these situations in the past. I am trying to remember that my reactions are stronger now because of my hormones. If I can be aware of that in the moment, I'm hoping it will give me a better perspective. It definitely takes practice."

Pretending that you are not experiencing a difficult emotion won't work in the long run, and it can make matters worse. So too can staying (too) busy as a means of avoidance. If you don't face uncomfortable emotions and deal with them in a constructive manner, they are bound to show up in unhealthy ways, whether that is overeating or acting impulsively. While it's important to engage in long-term stress-relieving activities (repeat after me: exercise!), sometimes you need a quick intervention to keep explosions at bay.

If you are feeling overwhelmed, try sitting still and breathing for a couple of minutes before you react. Concentrate on counting your inhalations and exhalations. Once your mind has stopped spinning,

Seven Ways to Deal with Brain Fog

While you may not be able to "cure" brain fog, there are ways to limit its effect on your work and personal life.

1. **Don't try to fake it.** It sounds obvious, but writing things down can be your salvation. If you have an important call or a presentation at work, put your thoughts on index cards or Post-its or in your phone, even if you used to be able to wing it. If you work with numbers and used to be able to do the calculations in your head, don't be embarrassed to reach for a calculator. Keep whatever tools you need handy.

2. **Stop multitasking.** While it is tempting to catch up on texts while watching TV or talking on the phone, multitasking impairs focus and memory.

3. **Get organized.** If you are having trouble remembering where you put your keys or your glasses, clutter isn't going to help. Create "safe spots" for your everyday objects: a hook by the door, a jewelry tray, a bin for shoes. Virtual clutter doesn't help either. Be sure to file emails into folders and flag those you absolutely must remember.

4. **CC yourself.** At work, ask people to email you with requests for meetings or important information rather than just saying it in passing. When sending notes or asking questions of others, cc or bcc yourself as a reminder.

5. **Use imagery and tricks to remember names.** Creating a mental image of a name or phrase can help with recall. For example, if someone tells you their name is Petra, try to picture a petri dish in the moment.

6. **Meditate.** Deep breathing and meditation are proven to reduce stress and anxiety, enhance performance on tasks, and improve overall cognitive performance.

7. **Prioritize sleep.** Sleep is the backbone of improved focus, mood stabilization, and pretty much everything else going on in your mind and body. Make sure you're setting aside seven to nine hours every night for some shut-eye.

acknowledge what you are feeling by pinpointing and naming it. Let's say you are disappointed with something your partner or coworker did. Acknowledge that and try to locate *where* you are feeling it. Is it in your heart? Your throat? Is there a tightness in your chest? After naming and locating the feeling, ask yourself, *Is it serving me?* If not, make a conscious decision to let go of it with your next exhalation. This exercise is not about suppressing a feeling but discovering a way to feel more in control of it so that you can deal with it at the appropriate time. Being able to identify what you are going through and explaining it in a calm moment to your partner, children, or friends can help them gain perspective and prevent even bigger blowups.

Along with stress, fluctuating hormones lead some women to have panic attacks, which can be accompanied by shortness of breath, dizziness, and heart palpitations.

Melanie Mills remembers that she was at her son's football game when she had the first panic attack of her life. "I had to walk across the bleachers to get to my seat," she remembers. "All of a sudden, something came over me and I was terrified that everyone would stare at me if I got up. I became absolutely paralyzed with panic, even though I knew it wasn't rational. I didn't tell my friend because I was sure she would think I'd lost my mind. I don't know how long I sat there, trying to think of different routes I could take back to my own seat. I've had fear of rejection in the past, but this was playing out in the weirdest way. I didn't tie it to my hormones until after the fact. Now if something like that happens again, I know enough to replace it with a more rational thought, which is, basically, 'No one cares about me crossing a field.'"

BUILDING BLOCK

Take a Belly Breath to Reduce Stress

You don't have to go to an ashram to get the benefits of meditation. You don't even have to sit still for a long period of time. Setting aside five minutes at the start and/or end of the day is a great way to get into the habit of deep diaphragmatic belly breathing, which can reduce cortisol (the stress hormone) and anxiety, lower your heart rate, and improve concentration within weeks.

To get the full effects of diaphragmatic breathing, Gabrielle Espinosa suggests this simple exercise. First, take a moment to notice where your breath is going. Do you feel it only in your upper chest? With the next breath, place your hands on your belly and imagine it ballooning out into your hands on the inhale and slowly deflating on the exhale.

These deep breaths put your parasympathetic nervous system, which controls your ability to relax, into what's called "rest and digest" mode, the calm state that follows a fight-or-flight response. After just a few minutes, you should feel the stress response in your body less and your mood improve.

Being aware of the possibility of hormone-induced panic attacks can remove some of the fear that accompanies them and spur preventive measures that decrease stress hormones and increase serotonin, including breath work, meditation, and exercise. If you continue to have panic attacks, speak to your doctor. Behavioral modification techniques and certain medications can help.

Lose the Labels and Find Out Who You Really Are

Taking the time to do a few psychological exercises can transform the moodiness of menopause into the impetus for growth.

Yes, you are moving away from the person you used to be, but if you are able to get past limiting notions of getting older, menopause can be life-affirming. When you are no longer defined by your reproductive capacities, you can look inside and connect with who you really are, recognizing your gifts, talents, wisdom, and all that you have to offer the world. Like any transformation, it can be confusing, painful, and frustrating at first, but there can be a sense of liberation when you come out the other side.

So many of us still have tapes playing in our heads that don't serve us. It could be something you heard from your parents, an ex-husband, or your employer telling you that you're not good enough. It takes work to let go of those tapes and replace them with a healthier belief system. The truth is, we don't have to be perfect, and we never actually will be.

It is not surprising that more women suffer from perfectionism than men. Many of us have been conditioned to take care of the people in our lives, excel at work, have a robust social life, and look good the whole time. Clinging to those impossible standards is bound to lead to low self-esteem, particularly during menopause when our bodies change, brain fog is real, and perfection is not an option. Guess what? It never really was.

Just ask Shania Twain. "Menopause taught me to quickly say, 'You know, it may only get worse,'" she told the *New York Post*. "'So just love yourself now. Just get over your insecurities—they're standing in your way.'"

Menopause can teach us to be more forgiving of other people as well as ourselves. Carol Mehas remembers working with older women who were going through the very changes she is now experiencing. "I hate to say it, but I realize now that I was very judgmental," she admits. "I feel terrible about that, but menopause has taught me to be more forgiving of others and myself. I've learned that you can actually gain more confidence when you let yourself give up on certain things. I found a greater sense of strength when I realized that it's okay if I can't wear a certain pair of pants anymore, or if I have to keep my notes handy during meetings. Accepting that has allowed me to move on and concentrate on other accomplishments that bring a sense of self-worth and make me feel valuable."

If you are struggling to let go of burdensome expectations, ask yourself these questions:

- **Are the goals you are setting for yourself realistic?** Are they *your* goals, or goals you *think* you should have?

- **Is fear of failure holding you back?** The idea that you have to be perfect at everything can keep you from trying new activities that might prove enjoyable. At this point in your life, you have probably failed at something. We all have. But the world didn't end. You got back up. That is how progress is made.

- **What narrative are you telling yourself?** We all tell stories about our lives, even if we don't publicly voice them. Are you telling yourself that you tried a new gym class and you fell off the equipment and felt like an idiot? Or are you telling yourself that you tried something new and it was hard, but you did it? Switching up how you think about an event can have a profound effect on mood and confidence.

Rediscovering Your Sense of Purpose

There is a huge shift taking place in our society. Ours is the first generation of women who are living to be ninety or even one hundred. That means we are also the first generation that is contemplating what our lives will look like in the second fifty years.

Menopause, like any major milestone, can be a time to take stock of where you have been, where you are now, and where you want to go. As life circumstances change, so too can your sense of purpose. Familial roles that occupied you in the past may be shifting. Perhaps you no longer feel the same passion for your career you once had. The sense of purpose that once propelled you may no longer feel relevant. Rather than a midlife crisis, what if you shifted your mindset and saw it as a midlife opportunity?

If you are a mother, you might start thinking about what your life will look like when caring for children is no longer one of your primary daily activities. If you are near retirement from your job, you might start thinking about who you will be when you no longer spend your days at work. The need for re-definition applies to all women, regardless of their family or relationship status. The question is: *How do I address the second half of my life?* The answer can't lie in anti-aging but in contemplating *how* you want aging to look and feel, and how you want to use your hard-won experience.

If someone asked you to say who you are in two minutes—the time of an "elevator speech"—could you answer them without using labels like "wife," "mother," "daughter," or your job title? Finding out who you are beneath those definitions will help you discover your truest self at this juncture in your life and align your actions to your values.

One technique that can help is to interview yourself as you would a stranger. Keep asking questions and peeling away the layers until you have your own personal elevator speech. Here are some prompts that can help:

- What do I want for myself?

- What brings me joy?

- What are my three biggest strengths?

- What are my values, my morals, and beliefs?

- Am I living by those tenets?

- What steps can I take to live in closer alignment with those tenets?

There are no right or wrong answers to these questions. You might have come up with social justice or forging deeper bonds of intimacy with your loved ones. You might want to try traveling on your own for the first time in your life. Dig into why those things are important to you.

There's no expiration dates for women. That has to go. Because you can kick ass at any age. You can hold your own at any age, you can dream at any age, you can be romantic at age. We have the right to be loved for who we are at the place that we are. We're not just here to make babies, we're not just here to baby the man. We're not just here to service everything and everyone around us and then when the kids go away . . . it's almost like expiration date for you as a woman. It's a misunderstanding that has been going around for centuries.

—SALMA HAYEK on *Red Table Talk*

The Importance of Social Connections

It can be tempting to withdraw from friends and social activities when you are not feeling your best. However, isolation not only makes you feel worse, but it may also increase the risk of cognitive decline and can lead to unhealthy behaviors, including drinking too much and overeating.

As a society, we are becoming more aware of the heavy toll social isolation and loneliness take. The U.S. surgeon general recently issued a report that found loneliness is far more than a bad feeling; it increases your risk of cardiovascular disease, dementia, stroke, depression, anxiety, and premature death.

The pandemic and its lingering aftermath caused many of us to get out of the habit of socializing face-to-face and led to an increase in social anxiety. Shying away from social connections can be a self-perpetuating cycle. The longer you go without that contact, the harder it can be to step out. Volunteering and joining a class can be good ways to ease yourself back into socializing. If there is a friend you have lost touch with, reach out. They may be feeling the same way.

For women going through menopause, social connections play another role. Because it is still not discussed in public as much as it should be, talking to other women can serve as a link to information and a reminder that you are not alone. There is nothing like another woman telling you that she forgot the name of her own pet to make you feel that you are in this together.

When Mary couldn't find a sense of community, she created one. "I felt really alone when I started going through menopause," she says. "I started a Facebook group for women who were also struggling. Creating a pocket of connection made a real difference. A lot of the things that we experience are scary, frustrating, or upsetting. We share the most embarrassing things, but knowing that there are other women going through similar things makes it less overwhelming."

I have found in my own life that having different circles of friends fulfills different needs. I have my closest friends, who I can be most vulnerable with. We can hang out and relax in ways I can't with many others. I have a group of high-achieving career women that I can talk about issues around balancing work and family life and hear how they deal with imposter syndrome. (Yes, I get it too.) I have mom friends for kid problems and friends I can turn to for financial advice when I need help strategizing. I have many colleagues in the field of women's health and nutrition (you've met some of them in these pages) with whom I share and compare findings. What all these groups have in common is a level of trust and support. That is the root of all true friendship. Take time to nurture your circle.

CHAPTER ELEVEN

Working through Menopause

Every woman's success should be
an inspiration to another. We're strongest
when we cheer each other on.

—SERENA WILLIAMS

Despite the fact that women are making huge strides in the workplace, menopause remains largely a taboo topic in offices, factories, and the service industry. The economic cost of continuing this silence to individuals, organizations, and society at large is stratospheric. A recent study done by the Mayo Clinic that followed more than four thousand women estimated the financial cost of missed workdays due to menopausal symptoms comes to $1.8 billion annually in the United States.

That same study found that 13.4 percent of women reported at least one adverse work outcome due to menopausal symptoms,

10.8 percent reported missing work in the preceding twelve months, and 5.6 percent reported cutting back on hours in the preceding six months. The reasons women gave included hot flashes, psychological symptoms, and urogenital issues. Similar research conducted in Britain found that a whopping 45 percent of women felt that menopausal symptoms had a negative impact on their work. There were even more women (47 percent) who needed to take a day off work due to menopausal symptoms but said they wouldn't tell their employer the real reason.

There are racial and ethnic differences here, too. Black and Hispanic women tend to have longer and more severe hot flashes than white women. Accordingly, the research found that higher percentages of Black and Hispanic women reported adverse work outcomes related to menopausal symptoms.

The personal stories behind numbers illustrate the true cost.

Lisa, forty-seven, a marketing executive in Pennsylvania, began getting hot flashes in her late thirties. "They were totally debilitating when I was at work," she says. "I would get very hot and sweaty for a couple of minutes. When it was over, I would be drenched. The air conditioning in the office made me shiver. I had to keep a fan on one side of my desk and a heater on the other. I avoided people because the hot flashes were so frequent and so unpredictable. When I worked from home, I avoided Zoom meetings because I didn't want people to see my face grow bright red. I finally went to my boss and said, 'You may have noticed a difference in my performance these past few months. I want to let you know that I'm having some medical issues, but I prefer not to speak about them.' I would love to see a world where women can be open and honest, but the work environment I'm in still puts an emphasis on being young. I was worried my managers would think I wouldn't be productive in the future. I didn't feel there was anyone I could go to."

Lisa is not alone in her reticence to speak up. In a recent survey of women in the workplace, over 80 percent of respondents said they had not spoken to an employer or manager at work about their menopausal symptoms. The reasons they gave include shame, fear of discrimination, and being seen as weak and making excuses.

Take a look at some recent statistics from a poll of 1,001 women in the UK. Perhaps you will recognize yourself in some of them.

- As many as 39 percent of women experiencing perimenopausal and menopausal symptoms are embarrassed to talk about it at work.

- Most women (60 percent) are in favor of additional menopause support from employers, but only 29 percent of women would feel comfortable asking for reasonable adjustments to support symptoms, such as an electric fan or flexible working hours.

- Less than half of women (49 percent) would feel able to raise a formal complaint if they felt they were being discriminated against as a result of experiencing menopause.

- Less than half of women (42 percent) feel comfortable taking time off work for menopause-related symptoms, and if they were to take time off, almost half of the women surveyed (48 percent) admitted they would lie about the reason.

- Many women (37 percent) said that menopausal symptoms would prevent them from re-entering the workforce if they were currently unemployed.

These numbers are unacceptable. As members of Generation M, we must fight against the stigmatization of menopause that threatens to hold us back financially and prevents society from benefiting from all we have to offer, just as we continue the fight against racism, sexism, and ageism.

Advocating for Change

Women going through perimenopause and menopause are usually in their forties and fifties, at the height of their earning power and their ability to contribute to companies' growth. If policies are not in place to support them, their career trajectories and lifetime financial security may be impeded, leading to further inequities at a time when women are still not treated equally in the workplace. The cost is not just personal. Businesses will miss out on women's brain and creative powers.

It would be nice to think all companies operate out of the goodness of their hearts, but highlighting the financial cost may be a more effective route to affecting change. Employee satisfaction and retention are important factors in organizations' success. Implementing policies that support the entire span of women's health can help to attract and retain talent.

Six Tips for Dealing with Hot Flashes at Work

1. **Keep a spare top at work.** Stash an extra blouse (and bra) in your bag or at your desk in case you need to do a quick change. Opt for natural fibers that absorb sweat and allow greater airflow to keep you cooler.

2. **Store cleansing wipes** for quick freshening-up, along with deodorant.

3. **Stash a small battery-operated fan** in your bag.

4. **Keep a ponytail holder handy** if you have long hair to get it off your neck.

5. **Try a cooling collar.** There are many discreet options that look (almost) like necklaces and freeze quickly to help cool you down.

6. **Get an instant ice pack.** These little packets freeze when you snap them so can be handily stored for when you need one.

Among changes that we can advocate for are increased training and education about menopause in the workplace, more supportive sick leave policies, and flexible work schedules.

These necessary accommodations are not beyond our reach. To put it into perspective, parental leave is a relatively new policy. Most workplaces didn't have pumping rooms for new mothers a

AMY'S STORY

I was drenched by the time I got to work.

The train ride to my job took about fifteen minutes but it felt like an eternity when I was in the middle of a hot flash. I had just showered, put on nice clothes, including a pressed shirt, and was rushing to a meeting. I would stress so much as I felt the beads of sweat on my face and heat emanating all over my body. By the time I got to work, I was drenched. I ran to the bathroom, washed my face, put a smile on, and tried to concentrate on the meeting rather than how bedraggled I was. On top of that, I was terrified I'd get another hot flash in the room and was obsessed with worrying that everyone was staring at me. It was so consuming, both physically and psychologically.

I was older than most of the women and our boss was a man. There was no one I could walk in to and say, "I'm having a hot flash." It was a culture where no one talked about things like that.

At first, I didn't want to take any drugs because I remembered stories about the cancer risk, so I just tried to deal with it. Finally, I connected with my OB/GYN, who referred me to a colleague in her practice who was well-versed in HRT. She was very candid about sharing her own experience, which made me feel better. I gained an understanding of the risks, which were very small for me. I really needed that support, because no one I knew was taking HRT then, or if they were, they weren't talking about it. I regret that I waited so long. I started feeling better very quickly and I am much less stressed at work.

—Amy, 52

decade ago. Mental health used to be a hidden issue in office settings. Accommodating menopause in the workplace is the next frontier in furthering women's health and economic equality.

Progress may be slow, but it is beginning to happen. Genentech, a biotech company with over 13,000 employees, recently instituted benefits that give women, their spouses, and partners access to menopause specialists, a drop-in menopause support group, and on-demand video chats and messaging with doctors, nurses, and coaches specializing in menopause, according to *Time* magazine.

If you need guidance for dealing with menopause in your workplace, the website The Hot Resignation has a downloadable toolkit with advice on how to review company policies, speak confidently to your HR representative, and advocate for change.

Take Control of Your Success Factors

While we work collectively to address how menopause is treated in the workplace, there are ways to improve your day-to-day experience now. Here are a few strategies to control your success factors at work.

- **Have a work ally.** A work ally is not a mentor but the one person you know will be in your corner and support you beyond your career trajectory. They don't have to be your best friend at work, and definitely shouldn't be someone who reports to you or you report to. Don't be shy about seeking someone out who you can go to when you are having a low moment or you're feeling uncomfortable in your own skin.

- **Know what does and doesn't help you.** Accept that your body—and your needs—are changing. Maybe you need to get more protein in your diet, or you find yourself getting hungrier at odd times. Keep healthy snacks in your drawer and a bottle of water handy. If you wear makeup, keep a kit in your desk drawer in case a hot flash makes it melt.

- **Learn to say no.** It's okay to set boundaries that reflect what you can and can't handle. It's not the amount of time but the quality of the work that matters. If you say yes to everything, you risk doing nothing well.

- **Don't be scared to use the crutches.** If you are worried about remembering numbers, have a calculator handy. Put thoughts on notecards for important calls or meetings. If you need reading glasses, use them!

- **Adjust what you can.** Ask for cooler temperatures or keep a fan nearby.

- **Take advantage of flexible work schedules.** If flexible hours or working from home some days is an option, start clocking when you tend to have low energy or brain fog and plan important tasks around that.

Generation M: Joining Forces for a Better Future

You must be the change you
wish to see in the world.

—MAHATMA GANDHI

There is nothing fiercer than when women band together for a common goal. That's what Generation M is all about. Defining ourselves. Advocating for ourselves. Making ourselves heard.

That means saying no to shame and yes to having a sense of humor. Because, trust me, I can pretty much guarantee you will morph into a burning inferno at least once at the worst possible moment. Remember my friend Deirdre who did a striptease in a restaurant? That's all of us. Laughing is by far the best option.

It means saying no to keeping silent and yes to talking openly about what we are going through. Menopause will never truly move out of the closet until we incorporate the people in our lives, including men, into the conversation. Who knows? Maybe one day my own mother will finally feel free enough to tell me what she went through.

It also means a hard no to being ignored and a strong yes to demanding answers from doctors and the medical community at large. This serves as fair warning to anyone who tries to patronize us.

It means absolutely no to a world where women's sexuality has an expiration date and yes to, well, whatever we damn please.

Finally, it means refusing to be defined by our reproductive viability and demanding respect for our vast capabilities.

Is that a lot to ask for? I don't think so.

We have come a long way from the time when perimenopause was barely acknowledged and menopause itself was treated as a form of madness. We are making progress from the days when women's health was relegated to an afterthought by the medical community and racial disparities were ignored or, worse, perpetuated. We are finally beginning to see wider acceptance of a holistic approach to health care that combines the best clinical research with proven mind-body practices, nutrition, and exercise.

But there is still a way to go.

I believe proudly waving the banner of Generation M can help get us there. Together, we can push past old narratives and create a new vision of women's health that promotes vitality across our lifespan.

Throughout these pages, you have learned the building blocks that can help you thrive through midlife and beyond. I encourage you to return to them over and over as you incorporate them into your daily life. Hopefully, you will be kind to yourself in the process. All sustainable habits take time to build. That is especially true when we are working to change not only physical behaviors but deeply ingrained mindsets as well. Every step you take, however small, is a step toward progress.

My vision for you—for all of us—is that we also focus on the building blocks that will help women everywhere feel empowered to speak up and demand access to information, treatment, and policies in the workplace that allow us to prosper.

As part of Generation M, we are lucky to have the second half of life to look forward to. If we prepare for it, support and advocate for each other, we will come to see perimenopause and menopause as natural rites of passage that lead to the next vibrant stage of our lives. Look out, world! We're on our way.

Notes

Introduction

xiv   *Recent studies have pointed out the large variations between African American, Hispanic, Japanese, Chinese, and Caucasian women when it comes to the severity of their symptoms and the treatment options they are offered*: Kimberly Peacock and Kari M. Ketvertis, "Menopause," in *StatPearls* (Treasure Island, FL: StatPearls Publishing, 2024), www.ncbi.nlm.nih.gov/books/NBK507826.

xvi   *Research published by the* British Journal of General Practice *shows that it takes ten weeks to build a new habit*: Benjamin Gardner, Phillippa Lally, and Jane Wardle, "Making Health Habitual: The Psychology of 'Habit-Formation' and General Practice," *British Journal of General Practice* 62, no. 605 (2012): 664–66, doi.org/10.3399/bjgp12X659466.

xviii   *the latest research also shows that as few as 3,000 to 4,000 steps per day can lower your risk of cardiovascular disease and overall mortality*: Maciej Banach, Joanna Lewek, Stanisław Surma, et al., "The Association Between Daily Step Count and All-Cause and Cardiovascular Mortality: A Meta-Analysis," *European Journal of Preventive Cardiology* 30, no. 18 (2023): 1975–85, doi.org/10.1093/eurjpc/zwad229.

Chapter 1
Your Roadmap: Where Are You Now? Where Are You Going?

4   *Talk to your doctor if you have four or more of these symptoms*: Nanette Santoro, "Perimenopause: From Research

to Practice," *Journal of Women's Health (Larchmont)* 25, no. 4 (2016): 332–39, doi.org/10.1089/jwh.2015.5556.

9   *Results from cross-sectional studies have indicated that the first endocrine changes characteristic of the onset of perimenopause may begin at around age forty-five*: Ellen B. Gold, "The Timing of the Age at Which Natural Menopause Occurs," *Obstetrics and Gynecology Clinics of North America* 38, no. 3 (2011): 425–40, doi.org/10.1016/j.ogc.2011.05.002.

9   *Average duration [of perimenopause]*: Nanette Santoro, Cassandra Roeca, Brandilyn A. Peters, et al., "The Menopause Transition: Signs, Symptoms, and Management Options," *Journal of Clinical Endocrinology and Metabolism* 106, no. 1 (2021): 1–15, doi.org/10.1210/clinem/dgaa764.

9   *Technically, natural (i.e., non–medically or surgically induced) menopause is a one-day event, indicating that you have gone twelve months without a period*: Pronob K. Dalal and Manu Agarwal, "Postmenopausal Syndrome," *Indian Journal of Psychiatry* 57, suppl. 2 (2015): S222–32, doi.org/10.4103/0019 -5545.161483.

9   *Hot flashes resulting from menopause last an average of 4.8 years for Japanese women, 5.4 years for Chinese women, 6.5 years for white women, 8.9 years for Hispanic women, and 10.1 years for Black women*: Nancy E. Avis, Sybil L. Crawford, Gail Greendale, et al., "Duration of Menopausal Vasomotor Symptoms Over the Menopause Transition," *JAMA Internal Medicine* 175, no. 4 (2015): 531–9, doi.org/10.1001 /jamainternmed.2014.8063.

Chapter 2
The Preseason: Perimenopause

13   *one billion women around the world will experience perimenopause by 2025*: Jan L. Shifren and Margery L. S. Gass, "The North American Menopause Society Recommendations for Clinical Care of Midlife Women," *Menopause: The Journal of the*

NOTES

North American Menopause Society 21, no. 10 (2014): 1038–62, doi.org/10.1097/gme.0000000000000319.

16   *It's estimated that 30 to 70 percent of perimenopausal women get hot flashes*: Santoro, "Perimenopause: From Research to Practice."

16   *The late transition is marked by at least two missed periods in a row*: H. Irene Su and Ellen W. Freeman, "Hormone Changes Associated with the Menopausal Transition," *Minerva Ginecologica* 61, no. 6 (2009): 483–89.

16   *Kelly Ripa shared her experience with this on her podcast*: Kayla Blanton, "Kelly Ripa, 53, Gets Candid About the Plus-Sides of Menopause," *Prevention*, October 9, 2023, www.prevention.com/health/a45455785/kelly-ripa-lets-talk-off-camera-podcast-menopause/.

17   *They are three times more common in Black women and two times more common in Hispanic women compared to white women*: William H. Catherino, Heba M. Eltoukhi, and Ayman Al-Hendy, "Racial and Ethnic Differences in the Pathogenesis and Clinical Manifestations of Uterine Leiomyoma," *Seminars in Reproductive Medicine* 31, no. 5 (2013): 370–79, doi.org/10.1055/s-0033-1348896.

19   *In fact, starting HRT during perimenopause not only can help lessen current symptoms, including hot flashes, mood swings, and trouble sleeping, but can also reduce their severity once you hit menopause*: A. A. Shargil, "Hormone Replacement Therapy in Perimenopausal Women with a Triphasic Contraceptive Compound: A Three-Year Prospective Study," *International Journal of Fertility* 30, no. 1 (1985): 18–28.

20   *starting HRT during perimenopause: It can reduce the chances of depression and combat vaginal dryness. It can help prevent osteoporosis and heart disease. And, if that's not enough, HRT's ability to help prevent Alzheimer's*

disease is strongest when it is begun during perimenopause: Howard N. Hodis and Wendy J. Mack, "Menopausal Hormone Replacement Therapy and Reduction of All-Cause Mortality and Cardiovascular Disease: It Is About Time and Timing," *Cancer Journal* 28, no. 3 (2022): 208–23, doi.org/10.1097/PPO .0000000000000591.

21   *Too little attention is paid to the emotional changes perimenopause can bring, including an increase in anxiety and depression*: Yuping Han, Simeng Gu, Yumeng Li, et al., "Neuroendocrine Pathogenesis of Perimenopausal Depression," *Frontiers in Psychiatry* 14 (2023), doi.org/10.3389/fpsyt.2023 .1162501.

21   *Isolation also puts you at greater risk for depression*: Morning Consult, "The Loneliness Epidemic Persists: A Post-Pandemic Look at the State of Loneliness Among U.S. Adults," Cigna Corporation, 2022, newsroom.thecignagroup .com/loneliness-epidemic-persists-post-pandemic-look. | Statement from the Office of the Surgeon General, "Loneliness in America."

Chapter 3
The Main Event and the After-Party: Menopause and Postmenopause

28   *Along with the immediate symptoms—hello, hot flashes—the loss of estrogen also has long-term implications*: Dalal and Agarwal, "Postmenopausal Syndrome," S222–32.

29   *The average age for its onset is fifty-one for white women in the United States and forty-nine for Black women. Hispanic and Native American women also tend to hit menopause earlier than white women, while Japanese women tend to go through menopause later*: Eun-Ok Im, Bokim Lee, Wonshik Chee, et al., "Menopausal Symptoms Among Four Major Ethnic Groups in the United States," *Western Journal of Nursing Research* 32, no. 4 (2010): 540–65, doi.org/10.1177 /0193945909354343.

29   *Many factors influence when menopause begins, including family history, genetics, weight, and lifestyle*: Ellen B. Gold, Gladys Block, Sybil Crawford, et al., "Lifestyle and Demographic Factors in Relation to Vasomotor Symptoms: Baseline Results from the Study of Women's Health Across the Nation," *American Journal of Epidemiology* 159, no. 12 (2004): 1189–99, doi.org/10.1093/aje/kwh168.

29   *Symptoms tend to be most prevalent and severe during the first one to two years*: Santoro et al., "The Menopause Transition: Signs, Symptoms, and Management Options."

32   *Women who have had their ovaries removed may have an increased risk of heart disease, stroke, cognitive impairment, and loss of libido*: Michelle Mielke, Ekta Kapoor, Jennifer R. Geske, et al., "Long-Term Effects of Premenopausal Bilateral Oophorectomy with or without Hysterectomy on Physical Aging and Chronic Medical Conditions," *Menopause* 30, no. 11 (2023): 1090–97, doi.org/10.1097/GME.0000000000002254.

33   *While 80 percent of women experience hot flashes at some point during menopause, certain factors influence when they start*: Nancy E. Avis, Sybil L. Crawford, Gail Greendale, et al., "Duration of Menopausal Vasomotor Symptoms over the Menopause Transition," *JAMA Internal Medicine* 175, no. 4 (2015): 531–39, doi.org/10.1001/jamainternmed.2014.8063.

33   *Smoking, drinking alcohol, a high-fat diet, and lack of physical activity can all contribute to turning up the heat*: Gold et al., "Longitudinal Analysis of the Association Between Vasomotor Symptoms and Race/Ethnicity Across the Menopausal Transition: Study of Women's Health Across the Nation," 1226–35.

33   *The Study of Women's Health Across the Nation (SWAN) is considered a hallmark of research into menopause in the U.S.*: Samar R. El Khoudary, Gail Greendale, Sybil L. Crawford, et al., "The Menopause Transition and Women's Health at Midlife: A Progress Report from the Study of Women's Health Across the Nation (SWAN)," *Menopause* 26, no. 10 (2019): 1213–27, doi.org/10.1097/GME.0000000000001424. | Gold et al., "Lifestyle

and Demographic Factors in Relation to Vasomotor Symptoms: Baseline Results from the Study of Women's Health Across the Nation," 1189–99.

34   *There are also racial and ethnic differences in how long symptoms last*: Ramandeep Bansal and Neelam Aggarwal, "Menopausal Hot Flashes: A Concise Review," *Journal of Midlife Health* 10, no. 1 (2019): 6–13, doi.org/10.4103/jmh .JMH_7_19. | Ellen B. Gold, Alicia Colvin, Nancy Avis, et al., "Longitudinal Analysis of the Association Between Vasomotor Symptoms and Race/Ethnicity Across the Menopausal Transition: Study of Women's Health Across the Nation," *American Journal of Public Health* 96, no. 7 (2006): 1226–35, doi.org/10.2105%2FAJPH.2005.066936. | Ellen W. Freeman, Mary D. Sammel, Jeane Ann Grisso, et al., "Hot Flashes in the Late Reproductive Years: Risk Factors for African American and Caucasian Women," *Journal of Women's Health & Gender-Based Medicine* 10, no. 1 (2001): 67–76, doi.org/10.1089 /152460901750067133.

35   *Unfortunately, 70 percent of women with moderate to severe hot flashes go untreated*: Rebecca Lee Smith, Lisa Gallicchio, Susan R. Miller, et al., "Risk Factors for Extended Duration and Timing of Peak Severity of Hot Flashes," *PLOS One* 11, no. 5 (2016): e0155079, doi.org/10.1371/journal.pone .0155079.

36   *Estrogen also plays a critical role in the brain's health and functionality*: Rebecca C. Thurston, Minjie Wu, Yue-Fang Chang, et al., "Menopausal Vasomotor Symptoms and White Matter Hyperintensities in Midlife Women," *Neurology* 100, no. 2 (2022): e133–41, doi.org/10.1212/WNL .0000000000201401.

37   *There is some evidence that eating soy-based products, which are rich in isoflavones, a phytoestrogen that mimics your body's estrogen, can lessen the severity of hot flashes*: Oscar H. Franco, Rajiv Chowdhury, Jenna Troup, et al., "Use of Plant-Based Therapies and Menopausal Symptoms: A Systematic Review and

Meta-Analysis," *JAMA* 315, no. 23 (2016): 2554–63, doi.org/10
.1001/jama.2016.8012.

37   *A diet consisting of mainly lean proteins, whole grains, fruits,
        vegetables, and olive oil, similar to the Mediterranean diet . . .
        may reduce the frequency and severity of hot flashes by up to
        20 percent*: Neal D. Barnard, Hana Kahleova, Danielle N. Holtz,
        et al., "A Dietary Intervention for Vasomotor Symptoms of
        Menopause: A Randomized, Controlled Trial," *Menopause* 30,
        no. 1 (2023): 80–87, doi.org/10.1097/GME.0000000000002080.
        | Gerrie-Cor M. Herber-Gast and Gita D. Mishra, "Fruit,
        Mediterranean-Style, and High-Fat and -Sugar Diets Are
        Associated with the Risk of Night Sweats and Hot Flushes in
        Midlife: Results from a Prospective Cohort Study," *American
        Journal of Clinical Nutrition* 97, no. 5 (2013): 1092–99, doi.org
        /10.3945/ajcn.112.049965.

38   *This is how clinicians define their severity*: Bansal and Aggarwal,
        "Menopausal Hot Flashes: A Concise Review."

39   *One study that followed over 1,000 women found that having
        negative beliefs about menopause*: Myra S. Hunter and Joseph
        Chilcot, "Is Cognitive Behaviour Therapy an Effective Option for
        Women Who Have Troublesome Menopausal Symptoms?" *British
        Journal of Health Psychology* 26, no. 3 (2021): 697–708, doi.org
        /10.1111/bjhp.12543.

39   *It can also lessen depression and improve overall quality of life
        during menopause*: Sheryl M. Green, Erika Haber, Randi E.
        McCabe, et al., "Cognitive-Behavioral Group Treatment for
        Menopausal Symptoms: A Pilot Study," *Archives of Women's
        Mental Health* 16, no. 2 (2013): 325–32, doi.org/10.1007/s00737
        -013-0339-x.

41   *The therapy is usually done with a therapist in thirty- to
        sixty-minute weekly sessions over a period of four to six
        weeks:* Myra S. Hunter and Joseph Chilcot, "Is Cognitive
        Behaviour Therapy an Effective Option for Women Who Have
        Troublesome Menopausal Symptoms?" *British Journal of*

Health Psychology 26 (2021): 697–708, doi.org/10.1111/bjhp
.12543.

42   *Menopause, with all its symptoms and uncertainties, can be
      stressful, but there are ways to feel more in control.* Nurdilan
      Şener and Sermin Timur Taşhan, "The Effects of Mindfulness
      Stress Reduction Program on Postmenopausal Women's
      Menopausal Complaints and Their Life Quality," *Complementary
      Therapies in Clinical Practice* 45 (2021): 101478, doi.org/10
      .1016/j.ctcp.2021.101478.

44   *numerous studies have shown that mindfulness-based and
      behavioral therapy can help alleviate perimenopausal and
      menopausal symptoms*: National Center for Complementary
      and Integrative Health, "Mind and Body Practices for Older
      Adults: What the Science Says," *NCCIH Clinical Digest for
      Health Professionals*, August 2019, www.nccih.nih.gov/health
      /providers/digest/mind-and-body-practices-for-older-adults
      -science. I Jennifer Britto John, D. Vinoth Gnana Chellaiyan,
      Sujata Gupta, et al., "How Effective the Mindfulness-Based
      Cognitive Behavioral Therapy on Quality of Life in Women with
      Menopause," *Journal of Mid-Life Health* 13, no. 2 (2022): 169–
      74, doi.org/10.4103/jmh.jmh_178_21. I Deborah Bowden, Claire
      Gaudry, Seung Chan An, et al., "A Comparative Randomised
      Controlled Trial of the Effects of Brain Wave Vibration Training,
      Iyengar Yoga, and Mindfulness on Mood, Well-Being, and
      Salivary Cortisol," *Evidence-Based Complementary and
      Alternative Medicine* 2012 (2012): 234713, doi.org/10.1155/2012
      /234713.

44   *One study of 1,744 women ages forty to sixty-five found that
      women with higher mindfulness scores had fewer menopausal
      symptoms*: Mayo Clinic, "Mindfulness May Ease Menopausal
      Symptoms," *ScienceDaily,* January 17, 2019, www.sciencedaily
      .com/releases/2019/01/190117090449.htm.

45   *The impact is greater for women who experience menopause
      before age forty-five*: Jiajun Liu, Xueshan Jin, Wenbin Liu, et al.,
      "The Risk of Long-Term Cardiometabolic Disease in Women

with Premature or Early Menopause: A Systematic Review and Meta-Analysis," *Frontiers in Cardiovascular Medicine* 10 (2023): 1131251, doi.org/10.3389/fcvm.2023.1131251.

46   *For women, a decrease in estrogen compounds these changes*: Kamila Ryczkowska, Weronika Adach, Kamil Janikowski, et al., "Menopause and Women's Cardiovascular Health: Is It Really an Obvious Relationship?" *Archives of Medical Science* 19, no. 2 (2022): 458–66, doi.org/10.5114/aoms/157308.

46   *The SWAN study found that the risk of heart disease varies across ethnic and racial groups*: Siobán D. Harlow, Sherri-Ann M. Burnett-Bowie, Gail A. Greendale, et al., "Disparities in Reproductive Aging and Midlife Health Between Black and White Women: The Study of Women's Health Across the Nation (SWAN)," *Women's Midlife Health* 8, no. 3 (2022), doi.org/10.1186/s40695-022-00073-y.

47   *In a study of 25,994 women in the U.S.*: Shafqat Ahmad, M. Vinayaga Moorthy, Olga V. Demler, et al., "Assessment of Risk Factors and Biomarkers Associated with Risk of Cardiovascular Disease Among Women Consuming a Mediterranean Diet," *JAMA Network Open* 1, no. 8 (2018): e185708, doi.org/10.1001/jamanetworkopen.2018.5708.

47   *hormone replacement therapy is proven to lower your risk of cardiovascular disease when given before the age of sixty and/ or ten years after the last period*: Suvarna Satish Khadilkar, "Post-Reproductive Health: Window of Opportunity for Preventing Comorbidities," *Journal of Obstetrics and Gynaecology of India* 69, no. 1 (2019): 1–5, doi.org/10.1007/s13224-019-01202-w.

48   *The American Heart Association (AHA) recommends 150 minutes of moderate exercise*: American Heart Association, "The American Heart Association Diet and Lifestyle Recommendations," Updated November 1, 2021, www.heart.org/en/healthy-living/healthy-eating/eat-smart/nutrition-basics/aha-diet-and-lifestyle-recommendations.

48   *A diet that includes fruits, vegetables, nuts, and limited processed food can lower your risk of heart disease*: Ibid.

48   *The Mediterranean diet, which includes fruits, vegetables, nuts, and olive oil and limits the amount of red meat and dairy, has been shown to lower the risk of heart disease*: Ibid.

48   *Diets high in sodium result in a 19 percent increase in heart disease*: Yi-Jie Wang, Tzu-Lin Yeh, Ming-Chieh Shih, et al., "Dietary Sodium Intake and Risk of Cardiovascular Disease: A Systematic Review and Dose-Response Meta-Analysis," *Nutrients* 12, no. 10 (2020): 2934, doi.org/10.3390/nu12102934.

49   *Ongoing and long-term loss of sleep can increase the risk of hypertension, high blood pressure, and cardiovascular disease*: Santoro et al., "The Menopause Transition: Signs, Symptoms, and Management Options."

49   *Slowing down your rate of inhalations and exhalations can reduce your heart rate, lower the risk of hypertension, and decrease stress*: Roderik J. S. Gerritsen and Guido P. H. Band, "Breath of Life: The Respiratory Vagal Stimulation Model of Contemplative Activity," *Frontiers in Human Neuroscience* 12 (2018): 397, doi .org/10.3389/fnhum.2018.00397.

50   *The Centers for Disease Control (CDC) found that one in four Americans over the age of sixty-five will fall*: Centers for Disease Control and Prevention, National Center for Injury Prevention and Control, "Older Adult Fall Prevention," Updated April 12, 2023, www.cdc.gov/falls/index.html.

50   *An estimated 50 percent of women over fifty years old will experience an osteoporosis-related fracture*: Tara Coughlan and Frances Dockery, "Osteoporosis and Fracture Risk in Older People," *Clinical Medicine (London)* 14, no. 2 (2014): 187–91, doi.org/10.7861%2Fclinmedicine.14-2-187.

50   *Falling once doubles the risk of falling again*: Coughlan and Dockery, "Osteoporosis and Fracture Risk in Older People."

NOTES

51   *The most common medications are bisphosphonates (for example, Boniva and Fosamax). These are generally the first-line treatment for osteoporosis and are quite effective, but bisphosphonates can have side effects*: William James Deardorff, Irena Cenzer, Brian Nguyen, et al., "Time to Benefit of Bisphosphonate Therapy for the Prevention of Fractures Among Postmenopausal Women with Osteoporosis: A Meta-analysis of Randomized Clinical Trials," *JAMA Internal Medicine* 182, no. 1 (2022): 33–41, doi.org/10 .1001/jamainternmed.2021.6745.

51   *The most serious, though rare, complication is osteonecrosis (bone deterioration) of the jaw:* Robert A. Adler, Ghada El-Hajj Fuleihan, Douglas C. Bauer, et al., "Managing Osteoporosis in Patients on Long-Term Bisphosphonate Treatment: Report of a Task Force of the American Society for Bone and Mineral Research," *Journal of Bone and Mineral Research* 31, no. 1 (2016): 16–35, doi.org/10.1002/jbmr.2708.

51   *Some patients also report gastrointestinal effects, such as acid reflux and esophageal irritation*: Adler et al., "Managing Osteoporosis in Patients on Long-Term Bisphosphonate Treatment: Report of a Task Force of the American Society for Bone and Mineral Research." Erratum in: *Journal of Bone and Mineral Research* 31, no. 10 (2016): 1910.

51   *One of the most effective is estrogen replacement therapy*: Dalal and Agarwal, "Postmenopausal Syndrome," S222–32.

52   *Along with working on your posture, improving the strength of your glute (i.e., butt!) and thigh muscles can protect your hip bones:* Robin M. Daly, Jack Dalla Via, Rachel L. Duckham, et al., "Exercise for the Prevention of Osteoporosis in Postmenopausal Women: An Evidence-Based Guide to the Optimal Prescription," *Brazilian Journal of Physical Therapy* 23, no. 2 (2019): 170–80, doi.org/10.1016/j.bjpt.2018.11.011.

53   *A few quick home exercises*: Anna Hafström, Eva-Maj Malmström, Josefine Terdèn, et al., "Improved Balance Confidence and Stability for Elderly After Six Weeks of a Multimodal Self-Administered

Balance-Enhancing Exercise Program: A Randomized Single Arm Crossover Study," *Gerontology and Geriatric Medicine* 2 (2016), doi.org/10.1177/2333721416644149.

53 *One activity that truly stands out for bone health and fall prevention is yoga*: Yi-Hsueh Lu, Bernard Rosner, Gregory Chang, et al., "Twelve-Minute Daily Yoga Regimen Reverses Osteoporotic Bone Loss," *Topics in Geriatric Rehabilitation* 32, no. 2 (2016): 81–87, doi.org/10.1097/TGR.0000000000000085.

54 *The Cleveland Clinic suggests these sources*: Cleveland Clinic, "Osteoporosis: Prevention with Calcium Treatment," Updated November 29, 2020, my.clevelandclinic.org/health/articles/15049 -osteoporosis-prevention-with-calcium-treatment.

55 *The thyroid is a small, butterfly-shaped gland in the front of your neck*: Rashmi Mullur, Yan-Yun Lu, and Gregory A. Brent, "Thyroid Hormone Regulation of Metabolism," *Physiological Reviews* 94, no. 2 (2014): 355–82, doi.org/10.1152/physrev .00030.2013.

55 *Because the thyroid is affected by estrogen levels, women are more likely to develop thyroid disease than men*: A. E. Schindler, "Thyroid Function and Postmenopause," *Gynecological Endocrinology* 17, no. 1 (2003): 79–85, doi.org/10.1080/gye.17.1 .79.85.

58 *Today, first-line treatment is usually monotherapy with levothyroxine, a synthetic form of T4 that your body converts to T3 and that is designed to mimic these hormones*: Wilmar M. Wiersinga, Leonidas Duntas, Valentin Fadeyev, et al., "2012 ETA Guidelines: The Use of L-T4 + L-T3 in the Treatment of Hypothyroidism," *European Thyroid Journal* 1, no. 2 (2012): 55–71, doi.org/10.1159/000339444.

58 *Every person converts T4 to T3 at different rates, and monotherapy may not address those differences*: Elizabeth A. McAninch and Antonio C. Bianco, "The Swinging Pendulum in Treatment for Hypothyroidism: From (and Toward?) Combination

Therapy," *Frontiers in Endocrinology (Lausanne)* 10 (2019): 446, doi.org/10.3389/fendo.2019.00446.

58   *Combination therapy in the form of desiccated thyroid extract made from animal thyroid glands is available:* Thanh D. Hoang, Cara H. Olsen, Vinh Q. Mai, et al., "Desiccated Thyroid Extract Compared with Levothyroxine in the Treatment of Hypothyroidism: A Randomized, Double-Blind, Crossover Study," *Journal of Clinical Endocrinology & Metabolism* 98, no. 5 (2013): 1982–90, doi.org/10.1210/jc.2012-4107.

58   *While these are not FDA-approved, they may be suitable for women who are not getting the desired results from synthetics or prefer a more natural alternative:* Sarah J. Peterson, Anne R. Cappola, M. Regina Castro, et al., "An Online Survey of Hypothyroid Patients Demonstrates Prominent Dissatisfaction," *Thyroid* 28, no. 6 (2018): 707–21, doi.org/10.1089/thy.2017.0681.

58   *As an added bonus, thyroid medications may also help menopausal symptoms and can be taken with HRT:* Ahmed Badawy, Omnia State, and S. Sherief, "Can Thyroid Dysfunction Explicate Severe Menopausal Symptoms?" *Journal of Obstetrics and Gynaecology* 27, no. 5 (2007): 503–5, doi.org/10.1080/01443610701405812.

59   *White Americans are twice as likely to be diagnosed with Hashimoto's disease:* Donald S. A. McLeod, Patrizio Caturegli, David S. Cooper, et al., "Variation in Rates of Autoimmune Thyroid Disease by Race/Ethnicity in US Military Personnel," *JAMA* 311, no. 15 (2014): 1563–65, doi.org/10.1001/jama.2013.285606.

60   *There are estrogen receptors all over your body that help to regulate insulin:* Monica De Paoli, Alexander Zakharia, and Geoff H. Werstuck, "The Role of Estrogen in Insulin Resistance: A Review of Clinical and Preclinical Data," *American Journal of Pathology* 191, no. 9 (2021): 1490–98, doi.org/10.1016/j.ajpath.2021.05.011.

NOTES

61   *HRT can significantly reduce the risk of metabolic syndrome
      and diabetes, especially when it is started early in menopause*:
      Nanette Santoro and John F. Randolph Jr., "Reproductive
      Hormones and the Menopause Transition," *Obstetrics and
      Gynecology Clinics of North America* 38, no. 3 (2011): 455–
      66, doi.org/10.1016/j.ogc.2011.05.004.

62   *Urinary tract infections (UTIs) become more common during
      menopause because the loss of estrogen lowers the vaginal pH*:
      Nicolas W. Cortes-Penfield, Barbara W. Trautner, and Robin L. P.
      Jump, "Urinary Tract Infection and Asymptomatic Bacteriuria in
      Older Adults," *Infectious Disease Clinics of North America* 31,
      no. 4 (2017): 673–88, doi.org/10.1016/j.idc.2017.07.002.

63   *Thirty-three million Americans are dealing with an overactive
      bladder*: Elad Leron, Adi Y. Weintraub, Salvatore A. Mastrolia,
      et al., "Overactive Bladder Syndrome: Evaluation and
      Management," *Current Urology* 11, no. 3 (2018): 117–25, doi
      .org/10.1159/000447205.

63   *thirteen million have urinary incontinence*: Linh N. Tran and
      Yana Puckett, "Urinary Incontinence," in *StatPearls* (Treasure
      Island, FL: StatPearls Publishing, 2024), www.ncbi.nlm.nih.gov
      /books/NBK559095/.

63   *81,000 are diagnosed with bladder cancer each year*: Rubab F.
      Malik, Renu Berry, Brandyn D. Lau, et al., "Systematic
      Evaluation of Imaging Features of Early Bladder Cancer Using
      Computed Tomography Performed Before Pathologic Diagnosis,"
      Tomography 9, no. 5 (2023): 1734–44, doi.org/10.3390
      /tomography9050138.

63   *Topical estrogen therapy in the form of tablets or creams can
      relieve urinary symptoms*: Bjarne C. Eriksen, "A Randomized,
      Open, Parallel-Group Study on the Preventive Effect of an
      Estradiol-Releasing Vaginal Ring (Estring) on Recurrent Urinary
      Tract Infections in Postmenopausal Women," *American Journal
      of Obstetrics and Gynecology* 180, no. 5 (1999): 1072–79, doi.org
      /10.1016/s0002-9378(99)70597-1.

Chapter 4
The ABCs of HRT

66   *However, in the years that followed, the WHI study was shown to have been deeply flawed*: Grace E. Kohn, Katherine M. Rodriguez, James Hotaling, et al., "The History of Estrogen Therapy," *Sexual Medicine Reviews* 7, no. 3 (2019): 416–21, doi .org/10.1016/j.sxmr.2019.03.006.

69   *The original goal of the research, which followed 27,347 women ages fifty to seventy-nine*: Angelo Cagnacci and Martina Venier, "The Controversial History of Hormone Replacement Therapy," *Medicina* 55, no. 9 (2019): 602, doi.org/10.3390/medicina55090602.

70   *The average age of the women in the study was sixty-three*: Katherine Machens and K. Schmidt-Gollwitzer, "Issues to Debate on the Women's Health Initiative (WHI) Study. Hormone Replacement Therapy: An Epidemiological Dilemma?" *Human Reproduction* 18, no. 10 (2003): 1992–99, doi.org/10.1093 /humrep/deg406.

70   *Further studies have shown that hormone therapy can significantly reduce the risk of cardiac disease*: Roger A. Lobo, "Where Are We 10 Years After the Women's Health Initiative?" *Journal of Clinical Endocrinology & Metabolism* 98, no. 5 (2013): 1771–80, doi.org/10.1210/jc.2012-4070.

70   *Plus, the study used only one type of synthetic progesterone*: John C. Stevenson, Serge Rozenberg, Silvia Maffei, et al., "Progestogens as a Component of Menopausal Hormone Therapy: The Right Molecule Makes the Difference," *Drugs in Context* 9 (2020): 2020-10-1, doi.org/10.7573/dic.2020-10-1.

71   *Most studies published since 2000 show that estrogen alone does not increase the risk of breast cancer*: Ronald K. Ross, Annlia Paganini-Hill, Peggy C. Wan, et al., "Effect of Hormone Replacement Therapy on Breast Cancer Risk: Estrogen Versus Estrogen Plus Progestin," *Journal of the National Cancer Institute* 92, no. 4 (2000): 328–32, doi.org/10.1093/jnci/92.4.328.

71   *The American Cancer Society has stated that in its view taking estrogen alone does not increase the risk of breast cancer*: American Cancer Society, "Menopausal Hormone Therapy and Cancer Risk," Updated February 13, 2015, www.cancer.org/cancer/risk-prevention/medical-treatments /menopausal-hormone-replacement-therapy-and-cancer-risk .html.

72   *The North American Menopause Society (NAMS) concluded*: Stephanie S. Faubion, Carolyn J. Crandall, Lori Davis, et al., "The 2022 Hormone Therapy Position Statement of the North American Menopause Society," *Menopause* 29, no. 7 (2022): 767–94, doi.org/10.1097/GME.0000000000002028.

73   *Certain supplements, including St. John's wort, ginkgo biloba, and melatonin, may interfere with how HRT is absorbed*: Katarzyna Zabłocka-Słowińska, Katarzyna Jawna, Halina Grajeta, et al., "Interactions Between Preparations Containing Female Sex Hormones and Dietary Supplements," *Advances in Clinical and Experimental Medicine* 23, no. 4 (2014): 657–63, doi.org/10 .17219/acem/37248.

75   *The study "Racial/Ethnic Disparities in the Diagnosis and Management of Menopause Symptoms among Midlife Women Veterans" was conducted by the Veterans Administration and followed 200,901 women*: Anna Blanken, Carolyn J. Gibson, Yongmei Li, et al., "Racial/Ethnic Disparities in the Diagnosis and Management of Menopause Symptoms Among Midlife Women Veterans," *Menopause* 29, no. 7 (2022): 877–82, doi.org /10.1097/GME.0000000000001978.

76   *Supplemental estrogen not only alleviates hot flashes and vaginal dryness, it can also protect against heart disease, inflammation, bone-weakening, and fractures due to osteoporosis*: Dalal and Agarwal, "Postmenopausal Syndrome." | Peter M. Tiidus, "Benefits of Estrogen Replacement for Skeletal Muscle Mass and Function in Post-Menopausal Females: Evidence from Human and Animal Studies," *Eurasian Journal of Medicine* 43, no. 2 (2011): 109–14, doi.org/10.5152/eajm.2011.24.

77   *Some studies have found the progesterone used in bioidentical*
       hormones has a lower risk of causing breast cancer than the
       synthetic hormones: Noor Asi, Khaled Mohammed, Qusay
       Haydour, et al., "Progesterone vs. Synthetic Progestins and the
       Risk of Breast Cancer: A Systematic Review and Meta-Analysis,"
       Systematic Reviews 5, no. 121 (2016), doi.org/10.1186/s13643-016
       -0294-5.

77   *Supplemental testosterone may improve sex drive, energy, and*
       overall well-being: Astrid M. Horstman, E. Lichar Dillon,
       Randall J. Urban, et al., "The Role of Androgens and Estrogens
       on Healthy Aging and Longevity," *Journals of Gerontology*
       (Series A, Biological Sciences and Medical Sciences) 67, no. 11
       (2012): 1140–52, doi.org/10.1093/gerona/gls068.

78   *A recent influential study in* JAMA *(*Journal of American
       Medical Association*) suggests that topical vaginal estrogen*
       may be safe for breast cancer survivors: Lauren McVicker,
       Alexander M. Labeit, Carol A. Coupland, et al., "Vaginal
       Estrogen Therapy Use and Survival in Females with Breast
       Cancer," *JAMA Oncology* 10, no. 1 (2024): 103–8, doi.org/10
       .1001/jamaoncol.2023.4508.

79   *Data regarding the effects of HRT on ovarian cancer is often*
       contradictory, but most studies show that HRT that contains both
       estrogen and progesterone can increase the risk: James V. Lacey Jr.,
       Pamela J. Mink, Jay H. Lubin, et al., "Menopausal Hormone
       Replacement Therapy and Risk of Ovarian Cancer," *JAMA* 288,
       no. 3 (2002): 334–41, doi.org/10.1001/jama.288.3.334. | Zosia
       Kmietowicz, "Short Term Use of HRT Increases Risk of Ovarian
       Cancer, Analysis Finds," *BMJ* 350 (2015): h840m, doi.org/10.1136
       /bmj.h840.

80   *Studies have shown that systemic HRT eliminates the symptoms*
       of vaginal atrophy in 75 percent of cases: Iuliia Naumova
       and Camil Castelo-Branco, "Current Treatment Options for
       Postmenopausal Vaginal Atrophy," *International Journal of*
       Women's Health 10 (2018): 387–95, doi.org/10.2147/IJWH
       .S158913.

80   *HRT increases calcium absorption and helps protect and strengthen bones*: Santoro et al., "The Menopause Transition: Signs, Symptoms, and Management Options."

81   *Researchers surmise that estrogen helps to protect against the deterioration of cognitive functions*: Délio Marques Conde, Roberto Carmignani Verdade, Ana L. R. Valadares, et al., "Menopause and Cognitive Impairment: A Narrative Review of Current Knowledge," *World Journal of Psychiatry* 11, no. 8 (2021): 412–28, doi.org/10.5498/wjp.v11.i8.412.

81   *The effects appear to be greatest when HRT is taken at the start of the menopausal transition*: Matilde Nerattini, Steven Jett, Caroline Andy, et al., "Systematic Review and Meta-Analysis of the Effects of Menopause Hormone Therapy on Risk of Alzheimer's Disease and Dementia," *Frontiers in Aging Neuroscience* 15 (2023): 1260427, doi.org/10.3389/fnagi.2023.1260427.

81   *Estrogen receptors help regulate insulin, the hormone produced in the pancreas that controls the amount of glucose in your bloodstream*: Saisai Li, Linjuan Ma, Yang Song, et al., "Effects of Hormone Replacement Therapy on Glucose and Lipid Metabolism in Peri- and Postmenopausal Women with a History of Menstrual Disorders," *BMC Endocrine Disorders* 21, no. 1 (2021): 121, doi.org/10.1186/s12902-021-00784-9.

81   *The increase in adipose (abdominal fat) common in menopause*: Morgana L. Mongraw-Chaffin, Cheryl A. M. Anderson, Matthew A. Allison, et al., "Association Between Sex Hormones and Adiposity: Qualitative Differences in Women and Men in the Multi-Ethnic Study of Atherosclerosis," *Journal of Clinical Endocrinology & Metabolism* 100, no. 4 (2015): E596–600, doi.org/10.1210/jc.2014-2934.

82   *In a study of over 56,000 women, HRT was shown to reduce the risk of colon cancer by up to 35 percent in postmenopausal women*: Jill R. Johnson, James V. Lacey, DeAnn Lazovich, et al., "Menopausal Hormone Therapy and Risk of Colorectal Cancer," *Cancer Epidemiology, Biomarkers & Prevention* 18, no. 1 (2009): 196–203, doi.org/10.1158/1055-9965.EPI-08-0596.

86   *The potential issues arise from the fact that compounded hormones are produced in individual pharmacies and are not subjected to the same tests for safety, efficacy, or dosing consistency as regulated HRT*: Louise Newson and Janice Rymer, "The Dangers of Compounded Bioidentical Hormone Replacement Therapy," *Journals of Gerontology (Series A, Biological Sciences and Medical Sciences)* 69, no. 688 (2019): 540–41, doi.org/10.3399/bjgp19X706169.

87   *The number of prescriptions of mostly unregulated compounded hormone therapy for women at menopause has reached an estimated twenty-six million*: JoAnn V. Pinkerton and Ginger D. Constantine, "Compounded Non-FDA-Approved Menopausal Hormone Therapy Prescriptions Have Increased: Results of a Pharmacy Survey," *Menopause* 23, no. 4 (2016): 359–67, doi.org /10.1097/GME.0000000000000567.

87   *One meta-analysis found that patients reported greater satisfaction with bioidentical hormones*: Kent Holtorf, "The Bioidentical Hormone Debate: Are Bioidentical Hormones (Estradiol, Estriol, and Progesterone) Safer or More Efficacious than Commonly Used Synthetic Versions in Hormone Replacement Therapy?" *Postgraduate Medicine* 121, no. 1 (2009): 73–85, doi.org/10.3810/pgm.2009.01.1949.

88   *a daily dose significantly relieved menopausal symptoms*: Kenna Stephenson, Pierre F. Neuenschwander, and Anna K. Kurdowska, "The Effects of Compounded Bioidentical Transdermal Hormone Therapy on Hemostatic, Inflammatory, Immune Factors; Cardiovascular Biomarkers; Quality-of-Life Measures; and Health Outcomes in Perimenopausal and Postmenopausal Women," *International Journal of Pharmaceutical Compounding* 17, no. 1 (2013): 74–85.

88   *Cardiovascular biomarkers, inflammatory factors, immune signaling factors, and health outcomes were favorably impacted*: Stephenson et al., "The Effects of Compounded Bioidentical Transdermal Hormone Therapy on Hemostatic, Inflammatory, Immune Factors; Cardiovascular Biomarkers; Quality-of-Life

Measures; and Health Outcomes in Perimenopausal and
Postmenopausal Women."

90   *Approximately one out of one hundred people experience side
effects from estrogen patches, gel, and spray*: National Health
Service, "Side Effects of Oestrogen Tablets, Patches, Gel and
Spray," Updated January 5, 2023, www.nhs.uk/medicines
/hormone-replacement-therapy-hrt/oestrogen-tablets-patches
-gel-and-spray/side-effects-of-oestrogen-tablets-patches-gel-and
-spray/.

91   *Approximately seventy-five percent of women who try to stop
are able to stop without major difficulty*: Deborah Grady and
George F. Sawaya, "Discontinuation of Postmenopausal Hormone
Therapy," *American Journal of Medicine* 118, no. 12, suppl. 2
(2005): 163–65, doi.org/10.1016/j.amjmed.2005.09.051.

91   *Studies have proven that acupuncture can help reduce hot flashes,
excess sweating, mood swings, sleep disturbances, and skin and
hair problems*: Kamma Sundgaard Lund, Volkert Siersma, John
Brodersen, et al., "Efficacy of a Standardised Acupuncture Approach
for Women with Bothersome Menopausal Symptoms: A Pragmatic
Randomised Study in Primary Care (the ACOM study)," *BMJ Open*
9 (2019): e023637, doi.org/10.1136/bmjopen-2018-023637.

Chapter 5
Will I Ever Sleep Again?

96   *Disrupted sleep activates the sympathetic nervous system and
affects the hypothalamic-pituitary-adrenocortical (HPA axis)*:
Alejandro F. De Nicola, Flavia E. Saravia, Juan Beauquis, et al.,
"Estrogens and Neuroendocrine Hypothalamic-Pituitary-Adrenal
Axis Function," *Frontiers of Hormone Research* 35 (2006):
157–68, doi.org/10.1159/000094324.

96   *Because both estrogen and progesterone help to regulate the
HPA axis, when they decrease, the HPA axis gets thrown off*:
Aviva Y. Cohn, Leilah K. Grant, Margo D. Nathan, et al., "Effects
of Sleep Fragmentation and Estradiol Decline on Cortisol in a
Human Experimental Model of Menopause," *Journal of Clinical*

Endocrinology and Metabolism 108, no. 11 (2023): e1347–57, doi
.org/10.1210/clinem/dgad285.

96   *The short-term consequences of sleep disruption for other-
      wise healthy adults can include increased stress*: Goran Medic,
      Micheline Wille, and Michiel E.H. Hemels, "Short- and Long-
      Term Health Consequences of Sleep Disruption," *Nature and
      Science of Sleep* 9 (2017): 151–61, doi.org/10.2147/NSS.S134864.

98   *Unfortunately, both natural aging and menopause itself cause
      melatonin levels to drop in most women*: Shazia Jehan, Giardin
      Jean-Louis, Ferdinand Zizi, et al., "Sleep, Melatonin, and the
      Menopausal Transition: What Are the Links?" *Sleep Science* 10,
      no. 1 (2017): 11–18, doi.org/10.5935/1984-0063.20170003.

99   *Acupuncture may also help to relieve hot flashes*: Huijuan Cao,
      Xingfang Pan, Hua Li, et al., "Acupuncture for Treatment of
      Insomnia: A Systematic Review of Randomized Controlled
      Trials," *Journal of Alternative and Complementary Medicine* 15,
      no. 11 (2009): 1171–86, doi.org/10.1089/acm.2009.0041.

99   *Extensive research has shown that practicing mindfulness . . .
      decreases sleep disturbances and improves the quality of rest*:
      Garrett Talley and John Shelley-Tremblay, "The Relationship
      Between Mindfulness and Sleep Quality Is Mediated by Emotion
      Regulation," *Psychiatry International* 1 (2020): 42–66, doi.org/10
      .3390/psychiatryint1020007.

101   *Not only is yoga one of the best forms of exercise for strength and
      flexibility, but it can also increase sleep quality and duration*:
      Mangesh A. Bankar, Sarika K. Chaudhari, and Kiran D.
      Chaudhari, "Impact of Long Term Yoga Practice on Sleep Quality
      and Quality of Life in the Elderly," *Journal of Ayurveda and
      Integrative Medicine* 4, no. 1 (2013): 28–32, doi.org/10.4103
      /0975-9476.109548.

104   *moderate exercise (think brisk walking) during the day can help
      reduce the time it takes you to fall asleep*: Alycia N. Sullivan
      Bisson, Stephanie A. Robinson, and Margie E. Lachman, "Walk
      to a Better Night of Sleep: Testing the Relationship Between

Physical Activity and Sleep," *Sleep Health* 5, no. 5 (2019): 487–94, doi.org/10.1016/j.sleh.2019.06.003.

105   *CBT is usually done with a therapist and takes about three to four weeks to be effective to improve sleep*: Matthew D. Mitchell, Philip Gehrman, Michael Perlis, et al., "Comparative Effectiveness of Cognitive Behavioral Therapy for Insomnia: A Systematic Review," *BMC Family Practice* 13 (2012): 40, doi.org /10.1186/1471-2296-13-40.

105   *In a study published in* JAMA Internal Medicine *that specifically targeted women with menopausal sleep problems, six CBT therapy sessions via telephone over an eight-week period improved sleep*: Susan M. McCurry, Katherine A. Guthrie, Charles M. Morin, et al., "Telephone-Based Cognitive Behavioral Therapy for Insomnia in Perimenopausal and Postmenopausal Women with Vasomotor Symptoms: A MsFLASH Randomized Clinical Trial," *JAMA Internal Medicine* 176, no. 7 (2016): 913–20, doi.org/10.1001/jamainternmed.2016.1795.

105   *Internet-based courses in CBT have also been shown to be effective*: Michael Seyffert, Pooja Lagisetty, Jessica Landgraf, et al., "Internet-Delivered Cognitive Behavioral Therapy to Treat Insomnia: A Systematic Review and Meta-Analysis," *PLOS One* 11, no. 2 (2016): e0149139, doi.org/10.1371/journal.pone.0149139.

107   *they are among the most prescribed medications in America*: Cynthia Reuben, Nazik Elgaddal, and Lindsey I. Black, "Sleep Medication Use in Adults Aged 18 and Over: United States, 2020," *National Center for Health Statistics Data Brief* no. 462 (2023), doi.org/10.15620/cdc:123013.

Chapter 6
Reclaiming Your Libido

114   *A large study published in the* British Journal of General Practice *found:* Alice Scott and Louise Newson, "Should We Be Prescribing Testosterone to Perimenopausal and Menopausal Women? A Guide to Prescribing Testosterone for Women in

Primary Care," *British Journal of General Practice* 70, no. 693 (2020): 203–4, doi.org/10.3399/bjgp20X709265.

114   *Doing Kegel exercises can help strengthen the pelvic floor*: María del Carmen Carcelén-Fraile, Augustín Aibar-Almazán, Antonio Martínez-Amat, et al., "Effects of Physical Exercise on Sexual Function and Quality of Sexual Life Related to Menopausal Symptoms in Peri- and Postmenopausal Women: A Systematic Review," *International Journal of Environmental Research and Public Health* 17, no. 18 (2020): 2680, doi.org/10.3390 /ijerph17082680.

117   *Getting moving (outside the bedroom) can increase activity in the sympathetic nervous system*: Amelia M. Stanton, Ariel B. Handy, and Cindy M. Meston, "The Effects of Exercise on Sexual Function in Women," *Sexual Medicine Reviews* 6, no. 4 (2018): 548–57, doi.org/10.1016/j.sxmr.2018.02.004.

117   *low levels of vitamin D have been associated with decreased sexual desire and pleasure*: Robert Krysiak, Małgorzata Gilowska, and Bogusław Okopień, "Sexual Function and Depressive Symptoms in Young Women with Low Vitamin D Status: A Pilot Study," *European Journal of Obstetrics and Gynecology and Reproductive Biology* 204 (2016): 108–12, doi .org/10.1016/j.ejogrb.2016.08.001.

121   *A meta-analysis of over 50,000 women found that alcohol reduces sensitivity to touch*: Nader Salari, Razie Hasheminezhad, Afshin Almasi, et al., "The Risk of Sexual Dysfunction Associated with Alcohol Consumption in Women: A Systematic Review and Meta-Analysis," *BMC Women's Health* 23, no. 1 (2023): 213, doi .org/10.1186/s12905-023-02400-5.

Chapter 7
Weight, What?

127   *Decreasing levels of estrogen shift how and where we store fat*: Seong-Hee Ko and YunJae Jung, "Energy Metabolism Changes and Dysregulated Lipid Metabolism in Postmenopausal Women," *Nutrients* 13, no. 12 (2021): 4556, doi.org/10.3390/nu13124556.

128   *Too much visceral fat can lead to metabolic syndrome*: L. M. Brown and D. J. Clegg, "Central Effects of Estradiol in the Regulation of Food Intake, Body Weight, and Adiposity," *Journal of Steroid Biochemistry and Molecular Biology* 122, nos. 1–3 (2010): 65–73, doi.org/10.1016/j.jsbmb.2009.12.005.

128   *Along with the specific health risks of visceral fat, being overweight in general can make menopausal symptoms, including cardiovascular risk, bladder health, and even hot flashes, worse*: Sakshi Chopra, K. Aparna Sharma, Piyush Ranjan, et al., "Weight Management Module for Perimenopausal Women: A Practical Guide for Gynecologists," *Journal of Midlife Health* 10, no. 4 (2019): 165–72, doi.org/10.4103/jmh.JMH_155_19.

131   *The most recent dietary guidelines for Americans recommend that healthy adults consume 10 to 35 percent of their calories a day from protein*: U.S. Department of Agriculture and U.S. Department of Health and Human Services, "Dietary Guidelines for Americans, 2020–2025," Ninth Edition, December 2020, www.dietaryguidelines.gov/sites/default/files/2020-12/Dietary_Guidelines_for_Americans_2020-2025.pdf.

131   *Studies show that eating less red meat can lower the risk of breast cancer in postmenopausal women as well as help to offset the heightened risk of heart disease*: Thais R. Silva, Karen Oppermann, Fernando M. Reis, et al., "Nutrition in Menopausal Women: A Narrative Review," *Nutrients* 13, no. 7 (2021): 2149, doi.org/10.3390/nu13072149. | Cody Z. Watling, Julia A. Schmidt, Yashvee Dunneram, et al., "Risk of Cancer in Regular and Low Meat-Eaters, Fish-Eaters, and Vegetarians: A Prospective Analysis of UK Biobank Participants," *BMC Medicine* 20, no. 73 (2022), doi.org/10.1186/s12916-022-02256-w. | Manuela Neuenschwander, Julia Stadelmaier, Julian Eble, et al., "Substitution of Animal-Based with Plant-Based Foods on Cardiometabolic Health and All-Cause Mortality: A Systematic Review and Meta-Analysis of Prospective Studies," *BMC Medicine* 21, no. 404 (2023), doi.org/10.1186/s12916-023-03093-1.

132   *Soy can be particularly helpful in reducing the frequency and severity of hot flashes*: Neal D. Barnard, Hana Kahleova,

Danielle N. Holtz, et al., "The Women's Study for the Alleviation of Vasomotor Symptoms (WAVS): A Randomized, Controlled Trial of a Plant-Based Diet and Whole Soybeans for Postmenopausal Women," *Menopause* 28, no. 10 (2021): 1150–56, doi.org/10.1097/GME.0000000000001812.

133   *Building Block: Ten High-Protein Foods to Add to Your Diet*: Johns Hopkins Medicine, "Protein Content of Common Foods," Updated June 2019, www.hopkinsmedicine.org/-/media/bariatrics/nutrition_protein_content_common_foods.pdf.

133   *As you get older, your body needs more protein to maintain lean muscle mass:* Masoud Isanejad, Joonas Sirola, Toni Rikkonen, et al., "Higher Protein Intake Is Associated with a Lower Likelihood of Frailty Among Older Women, Kuopio OSTPRE-Fracture Prevention Study," *European Journal of Nutrition* 59, no. 3 (2020): 1181–89, doi.org/10.1007/s00394-019-01978-7.

134   *Recent studies show that it may even help prevent cognitive decline*: Rocco Salvatore Calabrò, Maria Cristina De Cola, Giuseppe Gervasi, et al., "The Efficacy of Cocoa Polyphenols in the Treatment of Mild Cognitive Impairment: A Retrospective Study," *Medicina (Kaunas)* 55, no. 5 (2019): 156, doi.org/10.3390/medicina55050156.

134   *Reducing added sugar to below six teaspoons a day and limiting sugary drinks to less than one full serving a week can reduce the negative effects on your health*: Yin Huang, Zeyu Chen, Bo Chen, et al., "Dietary Sugar Consumption and Health: Umbrella Review," *BMJ* 381 (2023): e071609, doi.org/10.1136/bmj-2022-071609.

135   *As you get older, your metabolism slows, causing the sugar in alcohol to stay in your body longer:* National Institute on Aging, "Facts About Aging and Alcohol," Updated July 19, 2022, www.nia.nih.gov/health/alcohol-misuse-or-alcohol-use-disorder/facts-about-aging-and-alcohol.

136   *There's mixed evidence that suggests one glass of red wine per day may reduce the risk for cardiovascular disease:* Mariann R. Piano, "Alcohol's Effects on the Cardiovascular System," *Alcohol Research: Current Reviews* 38, no. 2 (2017): 219–41.

136   *It also increases the risk of weight gain*: Esra Tasali, Kristen
        Wroblewski, Eva Kahn, et al., "Effect of Sleep Extension
        on Objectively Assessed Energy Intake Among Adults with
        Overweight in Real-Life Settings: A Randomized Clinical Trial,"
        JAMA Internal Medicine 182, no. 4 (2022): 365–74, doi.org/10
        .1001/jamainternmed.2021.8098.

136   *When you are tired, there is a tendency to try to compensate for
        your lack of energy by upping your calorie (and sugar) intake*:
        Stephanie M. Greer, Andrea N. Goldstein, and Matthew P. Walker,
        "The Impact of Sleep Deprivation on Food Desire in the Human
        Brain," *Nature Communications* 4 (2013): 2259, doi.org/10.1038
        /ncomms3259.

136   *When you don't get enough rest, your body produces higher levels
        of ghrelin*: Tasali et al., "Effect of Sleep Extension on Objectively
        Assessed Energy Intake Among Adults with Overweight in Real-
        Life Settings: A Randomized Clinical Trial."

137   *Estrogen helps to maintain and regulate the energy balance in
        your body through the receptor ERα*: Fatemeh Mahboobifard,
        Mohammad H. Pourgholami, Masoumeh Jorjani, et al.,
        "Estrogen as a Key Regulator of Energy Homeostasis and
        Metabolic Health," *Biomedicine & Pharmacotherapy* 156 (2022):
        113808, doi.org/10.1016/j.biopha.2022.113808.

139   *Replacing estrogen not only can prevent weight gain but also has
        been shown to help in weight loss over a three-month period*: L.
        Chmouliovsky, F. Habicht, R. W. James, et al., "Beneficial Effect
        of Hormone Replacement Therapy on Weight Loss in Obese
        Menopausal Women," *Maturitas* 32, no. 3 (1999): 147–53, doi.org
        /10.1016/s0378-5122(99)00037-7.

140   *Studies have found that while this can lead to weight loss, it is
        likely due to the reduced calorie intake rather than some magic
        formula*: Ghada A. Soliman, "Intermittent Fasting and Time-
        Restricted Eating Role in Dietary Interventions and Precision
        Nutrition," *Frontiers of Public Health* 10 (2022): 1017254, doi
        .org/10.3389/fpubh.2022.1017254.

140   *Depression can lead you to self-medicate with food*: Yvonne H. C. Yau and Marc N. Potenza, "Stress and Eating Behaviors," *Minerva Endocrinology* 38, no. 3 (2013): 255–67.

144   *The Mediterranean diet has specific benefits for menopausal women*: Claudia Vetrani, Luigi Barrea, Rosa Rispoli, et al., "Mediterranean Diet: What Are the Consequences for Menopause?" *Frontiers in Endocrinology (Lausanne)* 13 (2022): 886824, doi.org/10.3389/fendo.2022.886824.

144   *Research indicates that it can improve the ratio of lean muscle mass to body fat*: Jadwiga Konieczna, Miguel Ruiz-Canela, Aina M. Galmes-Panades, et al., "An Energy-Reduced Mediterranean Diet, Physical Activity, and Body Composition: An Interim Subgroup Analysis of the PREDIMED-Plus Randomized Clinical Trial," *JAMA Network Open* 6, no. 10 (2023): e2337994, doi.org/10.1001/jamanetworkopen.2023.37994.

144   *A cross-sectional study in 481 postmenopausal women showed that a high adherence to the Mediterranean diet helped to reduce waist circumference*: Vetrani et al., "Mediterranean Diet: What Are the Consequences for Menopause?"

145   *The makeup of everyone's microbiome is different and is affected by age, diet, and genetics, as well as environmental factors*: M. Hasan Mohajeri, Robert J. M. Brummer, Robert A. Rastall, et al., "The Role of the Microbiome for Human Health: From Basic Science to Clinical Applications," *European Journal of Nutrition* 57, suppl. 1 (2018): 1–14, doi.org/10.1007/s00394-018-1703-4.

148   *The ensuing decline in hormone levels not only reduces this diversity and weakens your immune system, but it can also lead to a more permeable gut barrier*: Brandilyn A. Peters, Nanette Santoro, Robert C. Kaplan, et al., "Spotlight on the Gut Microbiome in Menopause: Current Insights," *International Journal of Women's Health* 14 (2022): 1059–72, doi.org/10.2147/IJWH.S340491.

148   *This allows bacteria and toxins to infiltrate the bloodstream, resulting in bloating, and in some cases, inflammatory bowel*

disease: Michael Camilleri, "The Leaky Gut: Mechanisms, Measurement and Clinical Implications in Humans," *Gut* 68, no. 8 (2019): 1516–26, doi.org/10.1136/gutjnl-2019-318427.

148 *An emerging body of research highlights the connection between gut health and brain function*: J. Horn, D. E. Mayer, Shelley Chen, et al., "Role of Diet and Its Effects on the Gut Microbiome in the Pathophysiology of Mental Disorders," *Translational Psychiatry* 12, no. 164 (2022), doi.org/10.1038/s41398-022-01922-0.

148 *Fiber helps maintain gut diversity and provides nourishment for beneficial bacteria*: Gijs den Besten, Karen van Eunen, Albert K. Groen, et al., "The Role of Short-Chain Fatty Acids in the Interplay Between Diet, Gut Microbiota, and Host Energy Metabolism," *Journal of Lipid Research* 54, no. 9 (2013): S2325–40, doi.org/10.1194/jlr.R036012.

149 *A short walk after eating can also speed up digestion*: Aidan J. Buffey, Matthew P. Herring, Christina K. Langley, et al., "The Acute Effects of Interrupting Prolonged Sitting Time in Adults with Standing and Light-Intensity Walking on Biomarkers of Cardiometabolic Health in Adults: A Systematic Review and Meta-Analysis," *Sports Medicine* 52 (2022): 1765–87, doi.org/10.1007/s40279-022-01649-4.

149 *Giving yourself a break from eating for up to twelve to fourteen hours may help your gut restore and replenish itself*: Falak Zeb, Xiaoyue Wu, Lijun Chen, et al., "Effect of Time-Restricted Feeding on Metabolic Risk and Circadian Rhythm Associated with Gut Microbiome in Healthy Males," *British Journal of Nutrition* 123, no. 11 (2020): 1216–26, doi.org/10.1017/S0007114519003428.

Chapter 8
The Exercise Rx

151 *Exercise can lower your risk of depression, ease anxiety, improve sleep, give you more energy, improve cognition, and boost your*

self-confidence: Laura Mandolesi, Arianna Polverino, Simone Montuori, et al., "Effects of Physical Exercise on Cognitive Functioning and Wellbeing: Biological and Psychological Benefits," *Frontiers in Psychology* 9 (2018): 509, doi.org/10.3389 /fpsyg.2018.00509.

152   *It may even help prevent Alzheimer's:* Helena Hörder, Lena Johansson, XinXin Guo, et al., "Midlife Cardiovascular Fitness and Dementia: A Forty-Four-Year Longitudinal Population Study in Women," *Neurology* 90, no. 15 (2018): e1298–305, doi.org/10 .1212/WNL.0000000000005290.

152   *According to the American Diabetes Association, exercise can lower your blood sugar levels for up to* twenty-four hours: American Diabetes Association, "Blood Glucose and Exercise," diabetes.org/health-wellness/fitness/blood-glucose-and -exercise.

152   *Exercise increases blood flow to the brain and improves executive function*: Ryan J. Dougherty, Stephanie A. Schultz, Taylor K. Kirby, et al., "Moderate Physical Activity Is Associated with Cerebral Glucose Metabolism in Adults at Risk for Alzheimer's Disease," *Journal of Alzheimer's Disease* 58, no. 4 (2017): 1089–97, doi.org/10.3233/JAD-161067.

152   *There are more brainy benefits: research shows that exercise improves neuroplasticity*: Arthur F. Kramer, Kirk I. Erickson, and Stanley J. Colcombe, "Exercise, Cognition, and the Aging Brain," *Journal of Applied Physiology* 101, no. 4 (1985): 1237–42, doi.org/10.1152/japplphysiol.00500.2006. | Mandolesi, et al., "Effects of Physical Exercise on Cognitive Functioning and Wellbeing: Biological and Psychological Benefits."

153   *Just twelve weeks of moderate exercise has been shown to improve vitality, mental health, and quality of life in menopausal women*: Jolanta Dąbrowska, Magdalena Dąbrowska-Galas, Magdalena Rutkowska, et al., "Twelve-Week Exercise Training and the Quality of Life in Menopausal Women—Clinical Trial,"

Przeglad Menopauzalny 15, no. 1 (2016): 20–25, doi.org/10.5114 /pm.2016.58769.

156   *Breaking that up with even short periods helps to counteract the negative health effect*: Chueh-Lung Hwang, Szu-Hua Chen, Chih-Hsuan Chou, et al., "The Physiological Benefits of Sitting Less and Moving More: Opportunities for Future Research," *Progress in Cardiovascular Diseases* 73 (2022): 61–66, doi.org/10.1016/j .pcad.2020.12.010.

159   *Combining these activities not only improves your physical well-being, but also has been shown to improve your memory more than aerobic exercise alone*: Greg Kennedy, Roy J. Hardman, Helen Macpherson, et al., "How Does Exercise Reduce the Rate of Age-Associated Cognitive Decline? A Review of Potential Mechanisms," *Journal of Alzheimer's Disease* 55, no. 1 (2017): 1–18, doi.org/10.3233/JAD-160665.

160   *studies show that strength training can also significantly reduce depression and improve body image in midlife women as well*: Brett R. Gordon, Cillian P. McDowell, Mats Hallgren, et al., "Association of Efficacy of Resistance Exercise Training with Depressive Symptoms: Meta-Analysis and Meta-Regression Analysis of Randomized Clinical Trials," *JAMA Psychiatry* 75, no. 6 (2018): 566–76, doi.org/10.1001/jamapsychiatry.2018 .0572. | Rebecca A. Seguin, Galen Eldridge, Wesley Lynch, et al., "Strength Training Improves Body Image and Physical Activity Behaviors Among Midlife and Older Rural Women," *Journal of Extension* 51, no. 4 (2013): 4FEA2.

160   *It may even help regulate hormone levels and lessen the impact of hot flashes*: Ana María Capel-Alcaraz, Héctor García-López, Adelaida María Castro-Sánchez, et al., "The Efficacy of Strength Exercises for Reducing the Symptoms of Menopause: A Systematic Review," *Journal of Clinical Medicine* 12, no. 2 (2023): 548, doi.org/10.3390/jcm12020548.

164   *High-intensity interval training (HIIT) is one of the most effective and time-efficient ways to improve heart health*: Muhammed Mustafa Atakan, Yanchun Li, Şükran Nazan Koşar, et al.,

"Evidence-Based Effects of High-Intensity Interval Training on Exercise Capacity and Health: A Review with Historical Perspective," *International Journal of Environmental Research and Public Health* 18, no. 13 (2021): 7201, doi.org/10.3390 /ijerph18137201.

165   *Mind-body workouts, including yoga and tai chi, can reduce the frequency and intensity of hot flashes and help you sleep better*: Kim E. Innes, Terry Kit Selfe, and Abhishek Vishnu, "Mind-Body Therapies for Menopausal Symptoms: A Systematic Review," *Maturitas* 66, no. 2 (2010): 135–49, doi.org/10.1016/j.maturitas .2010.01.016.

166   *the benefits can begin after just twelve weeks*: Purnima Madhivanan, Karl Krupp, Randall Waechter, et al., "Yoga for Healthy Aging: Science or Hype?" *Advances in Geriatric Medicine and Research* 3, no. 3 (2021): e210016, doi.org/10.20900/agmr20210016.

168   *The ancient form of exercise improves balance and bone density, and can enhance cognitive function*: Peter M. Wayne, Jacquelyn N. Walsh, Ruth E. Taylor-Piliae, et al., "Effect of Tai Chi on Cognitive Performance in Older Adults: Systematic Review and Meta-Analysis," *Journal of the American Geriatrics Society* 62, no. 1 (2014): 25–39, doi.org/10.1111/jgs.12611.

Chapter 9
Thin Skin, Thinner Hair

169   *During the first five years of menopause, though, your skin loses about 30 percent of its collagen*: M. Julie Thornton, "Estrogens and Aging Skin," *Dermato-Endocrinology* 1, no. 2 (2013): 264–70, doi.org/10.4161/derm.23872.

176   *Most topical solutions, whether serums or moisturizers, contain L-ascorbic acid*: Pumori Saokar Telang, "Vitamin C in Dermatology," *Indian Dermatology Online Journal* 4, no. 2 (2013): 143–46, doi.org/10.4103/2229-5178.110593.

181   *The actress Gabrielle Union opened up to* People *magazine about her menopausal hair loss*: Vanessa Etienne, "Gabrielle Union

Recalls Feeling 'Defective' Due to Perimenopause Hair Loss: 'Like Less of a Woman' (Exclusive)," *People*, November 17, 2023, people.com/gabrielle-union-felt-defective-due-to -perimenopause-symptoms-exclusive-8403678.

182   *foods rich in antioxidants can help skin stay supple and may reduce hair breakage*: Vivien W. Fam, Prae Charoenwoodhipong, Raja K. Sivamani, et al., "Plant-Based Foods for Skin Health: A Narrative Review," *Journal of the Academy of Nutrition and Dietetics* 122, no. 3 (2022): 614–29, doi.org/10.1016/j.jand.2021.10.024.

182   *Resveratrol can help fight the effects of sun damage, including discoloration and wrinkling, and aid in wound healing, and may even help slow or prevent skin cancer*: Kamil Leis, Karolina Pisanko, Arkadiusz Jundziłł, et al., "Resveratrol as a Factor Preventing Skin Aging and Affecting Its Regeneration," *Advances in Dermatology and Allergology/Postępy Dermatologii i Alergologii* 39, no. 3 (2022): 439–45, doi.org/10.5114/ada.2022.117547.

182   *Fatty fishes such as salmon have omega-3 fatty acids that help fight inflammation*: Céline Phan, Mathilde Touvier, Emmanuelle Kesse-Guyot, et al., "Association Between Mediterranean Anti-Inflammatory Dietary Profile and Severity of Psoriasis: Results from the NutriNet-Santé Cohort," *JAMA Dermatology* 154, no. 9 (2018): 1017–24, doi.org/10.1001/jamadermatol.2018.2127.

Chapter 10
This Is Your Brain on Menopause

184   *Nearly two-thirds of women report cognitive symptoms during perimenopause and menopause*: Gail A. Greendale, Arun S. Karlamangla, and Pauline M. Maki, "The Menopause Transition and Cognition," *JAMA* 323, no. 15 (2020): 1495–96, doi.org/10 .1001/jama.2020.1757.

185   *Estrogen receptors in various regions of the brain interact with the neurotransmitters responsible for mood, memory, and cognition*: Marques Conde et al., "Menopause and Cognitive Impairment: A Narrative Review of Current Knowledge."

186   *Eight weeks of aerobic exercise has been shown to increase both serotonin and endorphins*: Sayad Kocahan, Aykut Dundar, Muhittin Onderci, et al., "Investigation of the Effect of Training on Serotonin, Melatonin and Hematologic Parameters in Adolescent Basketball Players," *Hormone Molecular Biology and Clinical Investigation* 42, no. 4 (2021): 383–88, doi.org/10.1515/hmbci-2020-0095.

186   *Eating foods with magnesium and tyrosine, an amino acid, can boost dopamine production*: The Cleveland Clinic, "Dopamine Deficiency," Updated March 23, 2022, my.clevelandclinic.org/health/articles/22588-dopamine-deficiency.

187   *Certain techniques and behaviors like deep breathing and intentional focus . . . decrease stress, anxiety, irritability, and rumination*: Gerritsen and Band, "Breath of Life: The Respiratory Vagal Stimulation Model of Contemplative Activity."

189   *Approximately 20 percent of women experience some degree of depression during menopause*: Dalal and Agarwal, "Postmenopausal Syndrome," S222–32.

190   *Black Americans are twice as likely as white Americans to experience depression*: Nanette Santoro, C. Neill Epperson, and Sarah B. Mathews, "Menopausal Symptoms and Their Management," *Endocrinology and Metabolism Clinics of North America* 44, no. 3 (2015): 497–515, doi.org/10.1016/j.ecl.2015.05.001.

192   *Brain fog and memory lapses eventually plateau*: P. M. Maki and Nicole G. Jaff, "Brain Fog in Menopause: A Health-Care Professional's Guide for Decision-Making and Counseling on Cognition," *Climacteric* 25, no. 6 (2022): 570–78, doi.org/10.1080/13697137.2022.2122792.

192   *Hormonal changes can make existing cognitive conditions, including ADD and ADHD, more intense during perimenopause and menopause*: Evangelia Antoniou, Nikolas Rigas, Eirini Orovou, et al., "ADHD Symptoms in Females of Childhood, Adolescent, Reproductive and Menopause Period," *Materia*

Socio-Medica 33, no. 2 (2021): 114–18, doi.org/10.5455/msm
.2021.33.114-118.

193   *People who adhered to four to five of the following healthy
behaviors have a 60 percent lower risk of Alzheimer's disease*:
Klodian Dhana, Denis A. Evans, Kumar B. Rajan, et al., "Healthy
Lifestyle and the Risk of Alzheimer's Dementia: Findings from
Two Longitudinal Studies," *Neurology* 95 (2020): 1–10, doi.org
/10.1212/WNL.0000000000009816.

193   *As we get older, we have a heightened sensitivity to alcohol*:
National Institute on Aging, "Facts About Aging and Alcohol."

193   *Being intellectually engaged may help the brain become more
adaptable and compensate for age-related changes*: National
Institute on Aging, "Cognitive Health and Older Adults," Updated
October 1, 2020, www.nia.nih.gov/health/brain-health/cognitive
-health-and-older-adults.

197   *Deep breathing and meditation are proven to reduce stress and
anxiety*: Xiao Ma, Zi-Qi Yue, Zhu-Qing Gong, et al., "The Effect
of Diaphragmatic Breathing on Attention, Negative Affect and
Stress in Healthy Adults," *Frontiers in Psychology* 8 (2017):
874, doi.org/10.3389/fpsyg.2017.00874.

200   *It is not surprising that more women suffer from perfectionism
than men*: M. D. Musumeci, C. M. Cunningham, and
Theresa Leslie White, "Disgustingly Perfect: An Examination
of Disgust, Perfectionism, and Gender," *Motivation and
Emotion* 46, no. 3 (2022): 336–49, doi.org/10.1007/s11031-022
-09931-8.

201   *Just ask Shania Twain*: Chuck Arnold, "Shania Twain on Music,
Menopause and Loving Her Body 'More Now than Ever,'" *New
York Post*, September 13, 2023, nypost.com/2023/09/13/shania
-twain-on-music-menopause-and-her-sexy-future/.

202   *As life circumstances change, so too can your sense of purpose*:
Gabrielle N. Pfund, "Applying an Allportian Trait Perspective to

Sense of Purpose," *Journal of Happiness Studies* 24, no. 4 (2023): 1625–42, doi.org/10.1007/s10902-023-00644-4.

204   *There's no expiration dates for women*: Julie Mazziotta, "Salma Hayek Says Her Breasts 'Have Just Kept Growing' as She Goes Through Menopause," *People*, June 23, 2021, people.com/health /salma-hayek-says-her-breasts-have-just-kept-growing-as-she -goes-through-menopause/.

204   *isolation not only makes you feel worse, but it may also increase the risk of cognitive decline*: Santoro, "Perimenopause: From Research to Practice."

205   *The U.S. surgeon general recently issued a report that found loneliness is far more than a bad feeling*: Office of the Surgeon General, "Our Epidemic of Loneliness and Isolation: The U.S. Surgeon General's Advisory on the Healing Effects of Social Connection and Community," U.S. Department of Health and Human Services, 2023, www.hhs.gov/sites/default/files/surgeon -general-social-connection-advisory.pdf.

Chapter 11
Working through Menopause

207   *A recent study done by the Mayo Clinic that followed more than four thousand women*: Stephanie S. Faubion, Felicity Enders, Mary S. Hedges, et al., "Menopause Symptoms on Women in the Workplace," *Mayo Clinic Proceedings* 98, no. 6 (2023): 833–45, doi.org/10.1016/j.mayocp.2023.02.025.

209   *In a recent survey of women in the workplace, over 80 percent of respondents said they had not spoken to an employer or manager at work about their menopausal symptoms*: Biote, "Biote Women in the Workplace Survey," Updated May 10, 2022, biote.com /learning-center/biote-women-in-the-workplace-survey.

209   *Take a look at some recent statistics from a poll of 1,001 women in the UK*: Health & Her, "A Fact-Based Focus on Perimenopause

and Menopause Issues Faced by Women," 2019, committees
.parliament.uk/writtenevidence/39340/pdf/.

214   *Genentech, a biotech company with over 13,000 employees,
       recently instituted benefits that give women, their spouses,
       and partners access to menopause specialists*: Alana Semuels,
       "Now's the Time to Bring Up Menopause at Work," *Time*,
       June 29, 2023, time.com/6290706/menopause-care-work-us
       -companies/.

214   *If you need guidance for dealing with menopause in your
       workplace, the website The Hot Resignation has a downloadable
       toolkit*: The Hot Resignation, "The Hot Resignation
       Toolkit," hotresignation.com/hotresignation_toolkit.pdf.

Acknowledgments

There are countless people I would like to thank for the creation of this book. Throughout the writing process, just as in life, you realize how many people are a part of the fabric of your journey. I am extremely grateful to the incredible women who played an instrumental role in the creation of this book and shared their personal stories, experiences, and wisdom candidly. By sharing the moments of your life, from sweating profusely in public to starting a company devoted to prevention of health conditions, you bring power through your pain. This brings a depth of vulnerability and connection to menopause. To each of these remarkable women and my incredible sister, my sincere gratitude for your time and support.

Women physicians, scientists, and experts: this is our time. To shine, to focus, and to lead. So many women that contributed their expertise to the multifaceted dimensions of menopause have helped me broaden the commitment to advance and improve the lives of all women. Your dedication to advancing longevity and well span is truly inspiring. To Dr. Piraye Yurttas Beim, Dr. Christiane Wolf, Dr. Lisa Mosconi, Dr. Stacy Sims, Dr. Nan Wise, Dr. Melissa Mondala, Dr. Dendy Engelman, Tamar Samuels, and Hailey Babcock, your work not only inspires, it also brings a sense of solidarity among women in one of the most important times in their life.

ACKNOWLEDGMENTS

To my collaborating writer and editor, Emily Listfield, this story of menopause has many challenges and triumphs, and your keen eye, many calls, and tireless commitment to the production of this manuscript have given my words and ideas the chance to make it into the hands of many.

To my husband, Marvin, my parents, and my family, you know me at my best and my worst; thank you for allowing me to be me. Your encouragement and patience during this writing process has been substantial. I am grateful for your support.

Finally, to my little guys Chance and Miles, you are my inspiration in life. You show me every day that life is full of experiences and we have the ability to be present or not. This book was written in love through loud video games, making smoothies, towel fights after showering, and hugs with snuggles on the couch. Mama loves you.

Index

INDEX

INDEX

About the Author

Dr. Jessica Shepherd, a menopause expert and board-certified OB/GYN, is the recipient of numerous awards for her work as a physician and a leader in women's health. A thought leader in the field, she has been featured in *Forbes, Adweek, Vogue, Self, Women's Health*, and *MM+M*. She is a regular guest on *The Today Show, Good Morning America*, CNN, CBSN, and MSNBC.

As a nationally known health and wellness expert, Dr. Shepherd's practical and approachable strategies help individuals optimize their lives in their own way. With her extensive background in academia, Dr. Shepherd offers a fresh perspective on perimenopause and menopause, with tangible takeaways. She also challenges women to enhance their life outcomes and focus by helping them pay attention to what matters most in their lives.

Dr. Shepherd lives in Dallas, Texas, with her husband and two sons.